OTABIND®

 P9-CNA-022

Dear Friend:

You may have noticed that this book is put together differently than most other quality paperbacks. The page you are reading, for instance, along with the back page, is glued to the cover. And when you open the book the spine "floats" in back of the pages. But there's nothing wrong with your book. These features allow us to produce what is known as a detached cover, specifically designed to prevent the spine from cracking even after repeated use. A state-of-the-art binding technology known as OtaBind® is used in the manufacturing of this and all Health Communications, Inc. books.

HCI has invested in equipment and resources that ensure the books we produce are of the highest quality, yet remain affordable. At our Deerfield Beach headquarters, our editorial and art departments are just a few steps from our pressroom, bindery and shipping facilities. This internal production enables us to pay special attention to the needs of our readers when we create our books.

Our titles are written to help you improve the quality of your life. You may find yourself referring to this book repeatedly, and you may want to share it with family and friends who can also benefit from the information it contains. For these reasons, our books have to be durable and, more importantly, user-friendly.

OtaBind® gives us these qualities. Along with a crease-free spine, the book you have in your hands has some other characteristics you may not be aware of:

• Open the book to any page and it will lay flat, so you'll never have to worry about losing your place.

• You can bend the book over backwards without damage, allowing you to hold it with one hand.

• The spine is 3-5 times stronger than conventional perfect binding, preventing damage even with rough handling.

This all adds up to a better product for our readers—one that will last for years to come. We stand behind the quality of our books and guarantee that, if you're not completely satisfied, we'll replace the book or refund your money within 30 days of purchase. If you have any questions about this guarantee or our bookbinding process, please feel free to contact our customer service department at 1-800-851-9100.

We hope you enjoy the quality of this book, and find understanding, insight and direction for your life in the information it provides.

Health Communications, Inc.®

3201 S.W. 15th Street
Deerfield Beach, FL 33442-8190
(305) 360-0909

Peter Vegso
President

The '90s Healthy Body Book

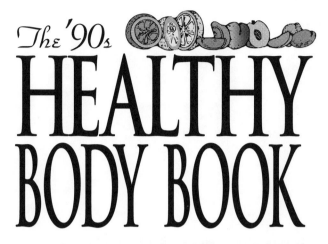

The '90s
HEALTHY
BODY BOOK

How To Overcome The Effects Of Pollution And Cleanse The Toxins From Your Body

Gary Null, Ph.D.

Health Communications, Inc.
Deerfield Beach, Florida

Library of Congress Cataloging–in–Publication Data

Null, Gary.
    The '90s Healthy Body Book : how to overcome the effects of
pollution and cleanse the toxins from your body/Gary Null.
        p.   cm.
    ISBN 1-55874-303-0
    1. Toxicology—Popular works. 2. Health. 3. Nutrition.
    4. Chelation Therapy. I. Title.
RA1213.N85 1994   94-1848
615.9—dc20   CIP

©1994 Gary Null, Ph.D.
ISBN 1-55874-303-0

Publisher: Health Communications, Inc.
               3201 S.W. 15th Street
               Deerfield Beach, Florida 33442-8190

Cover design by Robert Cannata

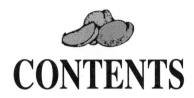

CONTENTS

Part Two: Cleansing and Rebuilding Your Body

SECTION V: Detoxification

Introduction To Life In A Toxic World

If you were to keep track, for even a few days, of all the toxins you encounter, how do you think the list would read? Chances are, it would look something like this: Automobile exhaust; industrial chemicals in indoor and outdoor air; contaminants such as industrial waste and farming chemicals in our water supplies; residues of fertilizers, pesticides and synthetic additives in "fresh" and processed foods; caffeine, alcohol and tobacco (both for those who smoke and those exposed to secondhand smoke); and potentially harmful ingredients in cosmetics and medicines.

What's wrong with this picture? Plenty. Why? Because it's only a broad sketch of our everyday exposure to harmful toxins. The reality is that we live in a toxic world, with pollution from multiple sources waging a sustained assault on our body systems. Our air, water, soil, food supply and household items all harbor health-threatening and sometimes carcinogenic chemicals. And our exposure to such toxins occurs in our homes, workplaces and neighborhoods. At the risk of overstatement, the pollution in our bodies has become a microcosm of the pollution in our personal environments. When we eat, drink and breathe toxins, we can be certain that our bodies are affected by them.

Of course, we have known about these poisons for some time. The devastating effects of pesticides on the environment and humans, for example, were laid out in Rachel Carson's groundbreaking book, *Silent Spring*, more than 30 years ago. But we have moved glacially, if at all, to control the very toxins that we know to harm us. The sale of pesticides has continued to climb since Carson wrote her book; they now poison more than 300,000 Americans every year and kill some 200,000 worldwide.[1]

These discouraging facts tell us that harmful and even deadly products continue to be used, despite the evidence of their ill effects on health. In the end, a product that is allowed to be sold will be sold. If fertilizers and pesticides are permitted on the market, they will continue to pollute our soil, water and food. If chlorofluorocarbons (CFCs) are permitted on the market, they will continue to deplete the ozone layer. If harmful industrial chemicals are permitted on the market, they will continue to pollute the environment. If antibiotics and other additives are permitted in the livestock-breeding process, their residues will continue to be passed to those who eat animal foods.

The message is that change must come from the top. While there's much to be said for individual and collective action to bring about positive change, ultimately it is our government and lawmakers who must see to it that the public health is protected from known carcinogens and damaging toxins. As long as the policy makers ignore the effects of these poisons—or wait for years, even decades, for "evidence" they should be curtailed or banned—the average citizen can do relatively little to avoid the large-scale poisons that pervade our environment.

The information in this book provides plenty of evidence that we are subjected to environmental poisons whose effects have been observed, measured and documented. It's time to stop making excuses and get change into effect. We need primary change, from the top, that removes toxins from our air, water, soil and food. We know what the problems are, and we know how they damage our ecosystems and the human body. Now we need a change in direction and meaningful solutions to recognized environmental dangers. It is my hope that this book will give you the impetus to get involved and demand change from your policy makers.

A Health Wake-Up Call

One thing is certain: What we don't know can hurt us. Take the chemicals that pollute our environment and bodies. More than 50,000 chemicals are in existence, and the Environmental Protection Agency (EPA) has estimated that 70 percent of these are a potential threat to the public health. Yet, only about 2 percent of these chemicals have been studied for all their effects on health, and the levels of less than three dozen of them are monitored in our drinking water.

Granted, the health of any one person is determined by many factors, including genetics, age, gender, diet and lifestyle. But as the pollution in our environment has increased, so has our incidence of illness and disease. And scientists are beginning to acknowledge that the possible link between the two cannot be ignored. Researchers in Sweden, for example, recently concluded a cancer study involving more than 800,000 people. They found that the cancer rate in men had increased 55 percent since 1958; in women, the increase was 30 percent. While cigarette smoking was the primary cause of cancer in the study, it did not account for the rising overall rates. Thus, the researchers said that cancer-causing agents in the environment were a possible cause.[2]

In the United States, too, the rate of death per 100,000 people with cancer has continued to rise over the past 50 years, increasing 19 percent between 1930 and 1989. And the increase in certain types of cancers—of the brain and prostate, melanoma and non-Hodgkin's lymphoma—is puzzling. In a recent interview with *Medical Tribune*, Aaron Blair, Ph.D., of the National Cancer Institute, stated: "You can't just explain it away with tobacco and better detection. None of these cancers has a large smoking component and for some, like non-Hodgkin's lymphoma, diagnosis is not a big issue. Occupational studies have revealed environmental exposures that may pose a hazard—exposures, such as lawn pesticides, which end up in the general environment."[3]

Also suspect is the standard American diet, which not only contains toxic substances but also is poorly balanced. We eat too many refined and processed foods, saturated animal fats and harmful products such as sugar and caffeine. Nearly all of the food we buy has been treated with chemicals and additives to "enhance" it in some way. That alteration means making it look or taste fresher, crisper and more flavorful than it naturally is. Our so-called "enriched" products have been stripped of their natural nutritional value in the production process, then loaded up with synthetic ingredients to mask their inferior quality.

The mass-production foods dominating our diet have little in common with those found in nature. The agitation, pressure and extreme temperatures used in processing can destroy the essential vitamins, minerals and amino acids contained in foods, making them much less capable of meeting the body's needs for these very nutrients. Vitamins such as C, A, D and E all can be lost in the refining process, for example, but food manufacturers may replace only some of these nutrients in the final product. And, of course, nutrients added to a denatured product can never achieve the nutritional balance of pure foods.

The safety and value of meat and dairy products have become especially questionable in recent years. While these animal foods provide us with protein, they also contain the residues of many potential toxins, including antibiotics, pesticides, hormones, preservatives and other additives. In some cases, they are also treated with nitrates and nitrites, substances known to contribute to the formation of powerful carcinogens in the body. And, despite the rampant use of antibiotics in livestock breeding, we have seen a rising incidence of illness and death from meat-borne pathogens, such as the *E. coli* and *Salmonella* bacteria. In fact, the widespread use of antibiotics has contributed to the development of resistant strains of bacteria that do not succumb to particular antibiotics.

Another harmful trend in the past few decades has been our increasing consumption of "fast foods." In the search for quick-and-easy meals, we have added another level of compromise to the quality of our diet. The meals served in fast-food establishments may be lacking in important nutrients, such as the B complex vitamins, but are high in dubious or harmful ingredients, including salt, preservatives, artificial colorings, sugar, fat and so on. Think of the standard fast-food fare: hamburger, bun, french fries and a milkshake or soda. All in all, a fatty, high-calorie meal with little nutritional value.

Given the multiple assaults on the body each day from toxins in our environment and the food supply, is it any wonder that our health deteriorates? Americans suffer from a slew of serious health disorders, including heart disease, cancer and other degenerative conditions. What's more, our immune systems have been weakened by the onslaught of foreign and toxic invaders, making us more susceptible to infections and diseases. We can no longer let these problems fester; the human and financial costs are simply too great. Life in a toxic world has not been kind to the individual, and it's time to make positive changes on our own—and demand the same from our policy makers.

PART ONE

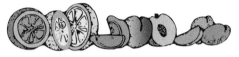

Our Toxic Planet Impacts Your Health

SECTION

I

Environmental Toxins

CHAPTER 1

Polluted Environment, Polluted Body

In recent years, Americans have finally started to face the grim realities of environmental pollution. It's not that we had much choice. Nature has let us know that the misuse and abuse of our air, water and soil will not go unnoticed. Today, the results of decades of environmental pollution are hitting home in all-too-alarming ways. Consider these facts:

- On a large-scale level, the industrial revolution has brewed up a heat-trapping mixture of carbon dioxide, nitrogen oxides, methane and chlorofluorocarbons (CFCs). The result is the "Greenhouse effect," a global warming that may cause extensive damage in the next century to farmlands, wetlands and beaches. At the same time, the ubiquitous CFCs are depleting the protective ozone layer of the earth's atmosphere, which blocks out cancer-causing and immune-weakening ultraviolet rays. And pollution-induced oxides are pouring down to earth in the form of acid rain, which destroys the ecosystem of our inland waterways.
- On a more immediate level, wanton pollution is having a direct impact on the public health. We breathe highly polluted air—

• indoors and out—which exposes us to toxic chemicals. We drink from water supplies contaminated with chemicals, pesticide residues and sewage. We eat food laden with harmful pesticides and chemical additives. And to top things off, we have a garbage problem. Our industrial and consumer waste is being dumped into landfills, where its toxic components can leak into the underground water supply, or burned in incinerators that produce a toxic ash. Our nuclear waste—containing such elements as plutonium and uranium—also is contaminating the environment.

In short, it's no longer possible to ignore the effects of pollution on the environment and our health. As pollution invades our homes and workplaces, each of us must take actions to reduce its consequences. While the Environmental Protection Agency (EPA) and the Food and Drug Administration (FDA) are responsible for protecting the environment and ensuring food safety, they have proved to be unreliable in carrying out those tasks. Pollution is a highly political problem, after all, involving powerful interests, including the chemical, drug, food and nuclear industries, to name just a few.

Despite their economic and political power, these industries cannot prevent us from seeking positive change. We can vote for politicians and support companies meeting our environmental ethics; we can change our consumption patterns to help prevent pollution. But first we need to educate ourselves about the pollution problems now plaguing this country. Consider the pages that follow to be a starting point in your quest for knowledge.

What's With The Air?

In the past few years, it has become increasingly clear that we cannot take the air we breathe for granted. Scientists around the world are sounding the alarm over air pollution, which has been taking its toll in disastrous ways. Three interrelated problems—global warming, ozone depletion and acid rain—threaten the balance of our entire ecosystem and expose us to health risks. Let's look at the factors behind these pollution problems:

Global warming. This environmental phenomenon generated national attention in the summer of 1988, when droughts caused more than one-third of our counties to be declared disaster areas. That's when the National Aeronautics and Space Administration's

(NASA) Institute for Space Studies informed Congress and the country at large that the Greenhouse effect does indeed exist. In essence, a variety of gases are creating a barrier that prevents the sun's heat from escaping into space. As a result, the global temperature may increase from three to eight degrees in the next 100 years—a significant change that can alter the planet as we know it.

By late 1988, the EPA had drafted a report predicting that global warming would have far-reaching and chaotic effects on the ecosystem. According to the report, the Greenhouse effect will have a damaging impact on our forests, farming system, the availability of water in our homes and workplaces, and the wetlands and beaches that supply us with fish and provide a source of recreation.

The culprits in global warming are four types of gases whose volume is increasing each year—carbon dioxide, nitrogen oxides, CFCs and methane. While carbon dioxide is the largest ingredient in the mix, the other three gases have greater heat-trapping capacities. CFCs (the ozone-destroying chemicals released by various consumer products) have 20,000 times the heat-trapping capacity of carbon dioxide; nitrogen oxides, a component of acid rain, have 250 times the capacity; and methane, released when organic matter decomposes, has 25 times the capacity.

Carbon dioxide is a naturally occurring gas that shouldn't be harmful when the ecosystem is in balance. But we have managed to make it a pollutant by releasing so much that its volume exceeds the earth's capacity to absorb and neutralize it. The burning of fossil fuels is a major contributor to carbon dioxide, whose concentration in the air has increased by about 75 parts per million (ppm) since the industrial revolution began. Of the more than 5 billion tons of carbon dioxide being released worldwide, about half can be absorbed by the oceans and forests.

Given that fact, the systematic burning of the tropical forests in the Amazon jungle is frightening. This massive destruction, which takes place through ritual annual burnings, may account for as much as one-tenth of the world's man-made output of carbon dioxide. It also diminishes the planet's ability to absorb carbon dioxide from other sources. The real tragedy is the driving force behind the destruction of the forests: to make room for ranchers who supply the American market with meat.

Automobile emissions are another big contributor to atmospheric carbon dioxide. They receive scant attention, however. That's because we would have to admit our dependence on the automobile is destroying the environment in order to address this problem head-on. But, like it or not, about 45 percent of our country's annual petroleum use is attributed to automobiles, which, in turn, account for more than half of the carbon dioxide found in our air.

Ozone depletion. It's easy to see why the thinning of the ozone layer is a crisis of huge proportions, and CFCs are largely to blame. This atmospheric layer, located 10 to 30 miles above the earth's surface, protects us from the potentially damaging effects of the sun's ultraviolet rays. By diminishing this protection, we expose ourselves to an increase in cancer, eye damage and other health ailments, such as a weakening of the immune system, and to the ultraviolet radiation of our wildlife, forests and crops.

One study in Australia found that air-pollution ozone levels may increase the risk of respiratory problems such as asthma in children. The study examined the effects of continuing exposure to the pollutant on more than 1,500 children ranging from 6 to 15 years old. Their respiratory risk was increased by ozone levels far below that the EPA considers to be safe.[1]

The news on ozone depletion keeps getting worse. In April 1993, NASA reported that the global ozone shield was at its thinnest ever in 1992, measuring 2 to 3 percent below previous readings. And preliminary measurements for 1993 showed that the ozone level over the Northern hemisphere was 10 to 20 percent below normal. The scientists speculated, but could not say for certain, that the unusually low ozone level was a temporary problem, caused in part by the impact of a mid-1991 eruption of a volcano in the Philippines. But even if that were so, the ozone levels would take a year or two to return to normal.[2]

The loss of ozone in the atmosphere has been tracked for some time now. The first major recording of the ozone layer's depletion took place in 1982, when scientists in the Antarctic discovered that the ozone layer had been reduced by about half its normal level at certain altitudes. Other scientists later identified ozone-layer reductions of as much as 97 percent at some altitudes in Antarctica.

The primary offenders in ozone depletion are CFCs, chemicals invented by E.I. DuPont Co. in the 1930s as "safer" replacements for a variety of chemicals used in consumer products. Over the years, CFCs have been used as coolants in refrigerators and air conditioners, foaming agents for the dashboards and seats in cars, propellants in aerosol-spray products (a use that was banned in the late

1970s) and cleansers for the circuitry of computer equipment.

By the mid-1970s, some American scientists were disturbed by the stability of CFCs—one of the chemicals' biggest selling points—and began to conduct research on them. They discovered that CFCs floated to the ozone layer, where the ultraviolet radiation of the sun caused them to break down into chlorine, fluorine and carbon. The exact mechanisms of how CFCs affect the atmosphere from that point on are still uncertain, but most scientists attribute the chemicals' ozone-damaging capacity to their chlorine component.

DuPont's response to the findings on CFCs has been a lesson in dithering and delay. The corporate giant, which controls nearly half of the United States' market for CFCs, began to develop CFC substitutes in the late 1970s. But this research effort came to a virtual standstill in 1978, when DuPont and other chemical makers realized that a regulatory ban on CFCs was not on the immediate horizon. Ten years went by before DuPont announced, in 1988, that it would discontinue its production of CFCs by the year 2000. This delay not only allowed tens of billions of pounds of CFCs to be released into the atmosphere, but also cost valuable time in coming up with alternatives.[3]

The question is, has the chemical industry's stalling put us so far behind that we cannot stop the forces we have unleashed? Even if CFC production is cut in half by the year 2000, the level of CFCs in the atmosphere may double within the next 50 years. In fact, an EPA study reported in the late 1980s that we would have to stop making CFCs—immediately and entirely—just to stabilize those already in the air.

Acid rain. The very concept of acid rain is enough to give anyone pause. Imagine that the by-products of our industrial lifestyle—sulfur and nitrogen oxides from coal-burning power plants, in particular, factory and automobile emissions and copper smelting—mix with precipitation in the atmosphere and then return to earth in rain, snow, fog or dust. That's exactly what happens with acid rain, which essentially pours an acidic solution into our lakes, farmlands, forests and oceans. The most common form of acid rain contains a sulfuric acid that results from sulfur oxide emissions.

When acid rain falls to earth, it causes major, long-lasting damage to freshwater lakes and streams. The poisonous acid alters the ecological structure of the water and its aquatic life. Bacteria and plankton, at the bottom of the food chain, are the first to die, followed by insects, frogs and fish. Eventually, the entire lake or stream becomes a dead zone. If the acid input were halted in a given lake, it might take as long as a century for the water to regenerate and return to its original state.

Acid rain is not a problem exclusive to the United States; this insidious pollution affects much of the industrialized world. But in the United States, the northeastern region has been particularly hard-hit. As long ago as 1982, a report by the Office of Technology Assessment showed that one-fourth of all lakes and streams in this region had been damaged by acid rain and thousands were endangered. The report concluded that acid rain was threatening the existence of as many as four-fifths of the lakes and streams in the Northeast and Upper Midwest.

Our coastal aquatic life also is susceptible to the ravages of acid rain. In this case, the damaging pollution results from nitrates and nitric acids, which are formed in the atmosphere from the nitrogen oxides produced by automobiles and electric utilities. These nitrates and other nutrients feed the algae in the ocean, causing a condition called eutrophication. In essence, the algae overgrows and cuts off the supply of oxygen and sunlight needed by other plants and animals.

Beyond that, acid rain affects our forests and even the buildings in which we live and work. According to a 1985 study of one portion of a mountain range in Vermont, for example, half the red spruce trees at high elevations had died in the previous two decades. Some experts believe this type of damage can be caused by pollutants that travel hundreds of miles from the industrial centers of the Midwest before they become an ingredient in acid rain. As for damage to buildings, another 1985 study estimated that acid rain caused about $5 billion worth of damage each year to houses and other structures in a 17-state region.

Until recently, the United States had a cavalier attitude toward acid rain. The issue was rarely discussed—let alone subjected to controlling legislation—until it started to make national headlines in the early 1980s. Even so, the United States chose not to ratify a 1985 proposal in which 16 countries agreed to reduce sulfur oxide emissions. The reason: We said we were doing enough already to control this type of pollution. Not until 1988 did we take a major step toward controlling the effects of acid rain. Then, along with two dozen other nations, the United States agreed to begin a program in 1994 to freeze the rate of nitrogen oxide emissions at 1987 levels.

Indoor Air Pollution

Before we leave the topic of air pollution, it must be noted that the air inside our homes and workplaces is highly suspect as well. Pollutants such as chloroform, formaldehyde and benzene proliferate indoors due to their use in paints, building materials, dry-cleaned clothes, cleansers and other products. In the workplace and at home, we may be exposed to the fumes that "outgas" from computers, copying machines, paint, carpeting and furniture. Toxins such as radon, carbon monoxide and asbestos also pollute indoor air.

There's no longer any doubt that these contaminants can have adverse health effects. In 1989, the EPA reported that indoor air accounts for a major portion of our exposure to pollution, and that the health risks posed by such pollutants can be serious and chronic. Depending on the individual involved and the severity of the exposure, indoor air pollution may cause anything from a runny nose to severe organ damage to cancer and death. In fact, pollutants such as radon, environmental tobacco smoke and volatile organic compounds pose significant cancer risks. What's more, the price tag for indoor air pollution is high, costing the country more than $1 billion a year in medical care.

Even so, only California, Washington and New Jersey have adopted indoor air regulations to date. In April 1993, New York also proposed an indoor air pollution bill that would establish the nation's strictest pollution standards. As reported in the April 23, 1993 edition of *Newsday*, the law would apply to all nonresidential buildings with more than 25,000 square feet of floor space.[4]

These buildings, whether public or private, would have to take one of two steps to reduce pollution: They could either circulate more fresh air in the building—at a rate of 20 cubic feet per minute per person—or take specific steps to clean up the building and reduce pollution sources such as chemicals and bacteria. State senator Michael Tully (R-Roslyn), the bill's sponsor and chair of the Senate Health Committee, told *Newsday*, "Plain and simple, nearly anyone who is in a building is subject to anything from Legionnaires' disease to asthma attacks to sickness of any kind. This is a big problem, and something needs to be done."[5]

Here's a summary of some major sources of indoor air pollution:

- *Carbon monoxide.* This gas can escape from a variety of appliances, including space heaters, furnaces and stoves, especially when they are not used and ventilated properly. Some 4.5 million people are exposed to carbon-monoxide levels that exceed federal safety standards, according to estimates from the National Center for Health Statistics. Carbon-monoxide poisoning from space heaters alone causes the death of about 200 people a year, and even one day of exposure to this gas, at the pollution level caused by some space heaters, can take a healthy person's blood level halfway to the point that causes nervous-system symptoms such as chronic fatigue and "brain fog," in which chemical reactions occur in the brain.

- **Radon.** In the late 1980s, the EPA pegged radon as one of the most serious environmental threats we face. This odorless and invisible gas is produced in the soil by deteriorating uranium. It then seeps indoors through the cracks of buildings, endangering hundreds of thousands of households. In fact, as many as 13,000 lung cancer deaths each year can be attributed to radon exposure, according to 1988 estimates from the National Academy of Sciences. And in a study of more than 10,000 homes in seven states, the EPA found that one-third had radon levels exceeding federal standards.

- **Formaldehyde.** This potent chemical is used in a wide variety of consumer products, including furniture components such as particle board, plywood paneling and medium-density fiberboard, certain fabrics, upholstery and carpeting, paper products and cosmetic items such as eye makeup and nail polish. Studies indicate that formaldehyde can cause cancer of the lungs, sinuses and liver. Although a federal safety commission banned the material's use in foam insulation in 1982 due to adverse health effects, a court later declared the ban to be invalid.

- **Volatile organic chemicals.** Many of our most common consumer products contain toxic chemicals that can damage the liver, heart and kidney, cause respiratory disorders and lead to bladder cancer. One of the most dangerous of these chemicals is benzene, a carcinogen found in paint and paint removers, dry-cleaning solutions and spot removers for clothing (which also contain the carcinogen toluene). Polishes, cleaners and shoe dyes contain dichlorobenzene, methylene chloride and trichloroethylene. Germicides and disinfectants contain cresol and phenol, a recognized carcinogen that can damage the central nervous system and various organs when absorbed through the skin.

Another solvent used to clean computer chips, called ethylene glycol ether (EGE), has been shown to increase the risk of miscarriage in female workers at two plants operated by IBM Corp. In a nine year study commissioned by IBM that ended in 1989, researchers found that women with high exposure to EGEs had a miscarriage rate of 33 percent; those with moderate exposure had an 18.9 percent miscarriage rate; and those who did not work with EGEs had a 14.9 percent miscarriage rate. The computer maker said it would phase out its use of the solvent by year-end 1994.[6]

• *Asbestos.* This insulating material was banned in the mid-1970s, when its ability to cause lung cancer was identified. In fact, asbestos causes of one of the worst forms of lung cancer, called mesothelioma, and a single fiber is capable of lodging in the lungs for years and eventually creating a tumor. Now, the United States faces the expensive task of removing asbestos from public buildings and schools.

However, it's not just chemicals, gases and the other pollutants that contaminate indoor air. Deadly bacteria also can get trapped in tightly contained and poorly ventilated buildings. In the infamous Legionnaires' disease tragedy in 1976, 29 people died at a Philadelphia hotel because bacteria had accumulated in the air-conditioning system. The victims inhaled the bacteria when it was distributed through the building by the cooling system. Similarly, a building's air may be contaminated by huge amounts of debris— from beer cans and food containers to dead insects and rats—that build up in the heating, ventilating and air-conditioning systems.

All of these contaminants contribute to the so-called "Sick-Building Syndrome," in which people become sick when they are exposed to chemicals, toxins and viral or bacterial agents indoors. In an effort to reduce energy consumption, many employers and landlords sealed up their buildings over the past few decades. Now, the resulting illnesses may be costing billions in medical expenses and lost productivity. Even so, the potential cost of restoring a building to environmental health may cause some employers and landlords to delay making positive changes or even deny that a problem exists.

The Water Of Life

Considering that water is necessary for survival, our treatment of it over the decades has been extremely shortsighted and negligent. We assume that anything we toss into our waters, be it garbage, untreated sewage or the toxic waste of industrial processes, will be diluted and detoxified by the vastness of the water systems. Not so. Water pollution has become an acute problem, destroying the ecology of one of our most precious resources and posing serious health risks to all forms of life, including plants, fish, animals and humans.

How have we managed to pollute such a wondrous and vital

resource as our waters? Here's a look at the factors at play:

Oceans. Recall the hot summer of 1993, when many of our country's beaches closed as a record-high volume of raw sewage, potentially infectious hospital waste and all-purpose garbage washed ashore. If that disastrous summer didn't convince us that we have a serious water-pollution problem on our hands, perhaps the following statistics will:

- Every day, at least 4.5 million metal containers are dumped into the sea, along with some 750,000 plastic and glass containers, by merchant vessels worldwide.
- Every year, the United States' commercial fishing fleet discards several hundred thousand tons of ropes, traps, buoys, packaging material and other plastics in the ocean. Navy vessels, recreational boats, cruise ships and offshore oil rigs also dump plastic garbage.
- The sediment in harbors nationwide is polluted with industrial chemicals, sewage and carcinogenic pesticides such as PCBs and DDT, which was banned from use in the early 1970s. The most highly polluted harbors are in Massachusetts, New York and New Jersey, while the San Pedro Canyon of California has the highest DDT level (a DDT maker dumped industrial waste in a Los Angeles harbor for years).
- Coastal cities around the world dump raw sewage into the ocean. And in some cities, the networks for storm drainage are linked with the sewer system. The result: Rainfall can dilute the sewage which then bypasses the sewage treatment facilities and is deposited in waterways.

In polluting the oceans, we endanger and kill marine animals which, quite literally, have nowhere else to go. Take, for example, Sylt Island in the North Sea, where fish with lesions and tumors have been found and where thousands of seals have died. Scientists suspect that pollution weakened their immune systems and made them susceptible to infections. Or we can look to our own backyard for the evidence of pollution's effects on marine life. In the late 1980s, hundreds of dolphins washed ashore in Florida and New Jersey, lobsters died all along the Long Island Sound, and thousands of dead fish, including crab, shrimp, flounder, bass and eels, washed up in New Jersey waters.

In addition to the dumping of waste, we also pollute our oceans with petroleum. The largest infusion of oil pollution comes from crude oil tankers flushing their tanks and discharging their ballasts at sea, according to research by the National Academy of Sciences and other organizations. In the North Sea, for example, an estimated 400,000 tons of oil are released each year by offshore oil rigs and ships. In Alaska, 13 million gallons of contaminated water are added to the sea each day by tankers. And a study of the Gulf of Mexico has found it to be one of the world's most polluted bodies of water.

And then, of course, the ocean is polluted by oil spills, such as the three that occurred in rapid succession in late 1988 and early 1989. In Alaska's Prince William Sound, the Exxon Valdez spilled tens of millions of gallons of crude oil; in Grays Harbor in Washington state, hundreds of thousands of gallons were spilled; and near the Antarctic Peninsula, a ship began leaking about 3,000 gallons of fuel and crude oil a day.

With the Exxon oil spill alone, the largest in U.S. history, enormous damage was done to the environment. Exxon's ability to contain such a spill was grossly inadequate, and the oil spread for several days before any major steps were taken to control it. The crude oil, which contains poisonous, carcinogenic substances, blanketed the area's animal life. Sea otters were nearly frozen because crude oil on their fur interfered with its insulating ability. And for every 100 yards of beach, an average of more than 80 ducks and other birds were found covered with oil.

Rivers and inland waters. Many of our rivers, lakes and streams have been so fouled by sewage, garbage and industrial waste during the past century that we have, in a sense, turned our backs on them and put them out of our minds. Only when something extraordinary happens—say, when the Cuyahoga River running from Lake Erie to Cleveland literally caught fire in 1968—do we face the fact that the condition of our waters is causing extensive environmental damage.

The polluting of our waters with chemicals has increased tremendously since World War II, when we began to produce massive quantities of synthetic chemicals, solvents and plastics. Petrochemicals, the byproducts of oil refining, serve as a base for many synthetic chemicals, and the lion's share of our chemical pollution today can be attributed to the petrochemical industry. Now 60 percent of our hazardous waste is caused by chemical production.

What's alarming is how little we know about the chemicals already in existence—which now number more than 50,000. To this lengthy list, another 1,000 or so new chemicals are added each year. The chemical industry, in typical fashion, reveals nothing of the properties of chemicals being dumped into our waters. But the EPA has estimated that more than two-thirds of all chemicals—a staggering 35,000 compounds—pose a threat to human health.

The evidence of these chemicals' effects can be found in the fish in our rivers and lakes. The health of these fish and other aquatic life is a good indication of whether an ecosystem is in balance; when they suffer, we can extrapolate that the ecological imbalance eventually will affect humans as well. A case in point: The effects of dioxin, a chemical used by paper mills to bleach paper, were first discovered because eggshells were unnaturally soft. Scientists researched the areas in which fish were dying of cancer and found that the incidence of cancer in humans was unusually high as well.

Indeed, freshwater fish have suffered from an epidemic of skin and liver cancer in five areas of the United States near industrial centers. In 1983, all saucer pike at one Michigan site were hit with a cancer epidemic. And in 1987, the Michigan Department of Natural Resources found that various birds feeding on fish in the Great Lakes had reproductive failures and birth defects. Lake Erie, in particular, has been so polluted for so long that as early as 1953 magpies could no longer hatch on its surface.

Chemical pollution is a widespread problem, leaving few of our large bodies of water unaffected. In a 1989 study of dioxin the EPA found that fish located downstream from one-fourth of the 81 paper mills studied had dioxin levels exceeding the federal hazardous point. In fact, they had seven times as much dioxin as the level considered dangerous for human consumption by the FDA. Dioxin is a known carcinogen—and a component of Agent Orange, a chemical defoliant used in the war in Vietnam that can cause a skin condition called chloracne and lead to immune system damage.

Drinking water. As the residents of Milwaukee and surrounding communities discovered in early 1993, the safety of our drinking water is far from guaranteed. Due to a failure in the area's water-purification and filtering system, some 200,000 people were stricken with an illness caused by *cryptosporidium*, a feces-transmitted parasite that sets up shop in the intestines and causes diarrhea, cramping and vomiting until the immune system can get the invader under control.

The Milwaukee outbreak reminded the nation, yet again, that

our community water systems are susceptible to contamination from a variety of fronts—including bacteria, viruses and parasites, and also chemical pollutants, pesticides and even nuclear waste. To make matters worse, many of our nearly 200,000 water systems, either community-based or smaller, are aging and poorly run. As reported in the *New York Times*, the General Accounting Office (GAO) issued a report in April 1993 criticizing the status of state water-inspection programs. Said the *Times*: "[The report] found that most state inspection programs to ensure the safety of public water supplies are a shambles."[7]

The EPA recommends that states inspect their water at least once every three years, but 26 states had not done so according to the GAO report. In fact, some water systems have not been inspected in more than a decade, which means the drinking water supplied to the public could have "significant undetected deficiencies." What's more, deficiencies detected may not be corrected. "The report cited as the most frequent problem the lack of programs to ensure that drinking water not become mixed with contaminated water and sewage," the *Times* stated.[8]

But parasites and microbes are not the only contaminants in our waterworks. In 1982, the EPA found organic chemicals in 45 percent of the underground aquifers supplying large public water systems. Across the country in places like Ohio, New Jersey, New York, California, Washington, Texas and South Carolina the water tables have been polluted with chemicals, pesticides and radioactive waste. More than half of the nation's drinking water is being polluted by leaking hazardous-waste sites.

Unfortunately, our government does very little to protect us from such disease-causing contaminants. Of the 50,000 chemicals on the market, the EPA regulates the level of 30 of them in our drinking water; only about 500 chemicals have been analyzed for cancer-causing properties. Nor does the government give much attention to enforcing the Safe Drinking Water Act. In late 1988, the National Wildlife Federation issued a report charging that the law was violated more than 100,000 times in 1987 by public water systems supplying 36 million Americans. The states acted on these violations less than 2,600 times; the EPA took action in a mere 50 cases.

The toxic chemicals now polluting our water supplies include the following:

• *Benzene.* Industrial waste, agricultural runoff and leaky fuel tanks deposit this petroleum-based liquid in our water supplies. Benzene is a carcinogenic ingredient of paints, pesticides, plastics, detergents and pharmaceuticals. It's also a chemical component of gasoline, which now pollutes about 40 percent of the country's groundwater. Of our 2.5 million gasoline storage tanks, in fact, nearly one-fourth may be leaking, according to EPA estimates. And the benzene contained in only one gallon of gasoline can contaminate 75,000 gallons of water.

- *Trichloroethylene (TCE).* Even small amounts of this chemical, contained in pesticides, grease removers, paints, varnishes and strippers, are suspected of causing cancer. The level of TCE in drinking water can reach dangerously high levels. In the early 1980s, the TCE level was 18 times above federal safety standards in Des Moines, Iowa, where a company used the product in the 1960s and then dumped it down the drain. And in Fort Edwards, New York, the TCE level soared to 2,000 times the standard due to leakage from a General Electric factory.

- *Polychlorinated biphenyls (PCBs).* These chemicals include extremely toxic substances such as DDT and dioxin (TCDD), both of which share certain properties with the ozone-damaging CFCs. These chlorine derivatives are stable, durable, nonconducting and nonflammable. As such, manufacturers use them in plastics, paints, sealers, pesticides, electrical equipment such as transformers and heat-exchanger fluids. They end up in our drinking water via sewage and industrial waste.

  It is estimated that up to 80 percent of the world's people have measurable levels of PCBs in their bodies, yet the EPA does not include these chemicals among the 30 it regulates in drinking water. Dioxin, in particular, is one of the most toxic chemicals in existence. It can be fatal at concentrations as low as 1 part per billion, and at even lower levels it can cause skin rashes, systemic disorders and even cancer. Although dioxin often is emitted by paper mills that produce it as a by-product when they bleach paper with chlorine, traces of the chemical are hard to detect because of its highly toxic nature. The only sure way to protect the population from this lethal substance is to ban dioxin emissions entirely.

- *Inorganic chemicals.* This family of chemicals includes arsenic, lead, barium, cadmium and chromium, all of which end up in the water supply and lead to adverse health effects. Arsenic and barium, for example, contaminate our waters via industrial waste, pesticide residue and smelting operations. Arsenic can damage the nervous system and cause skin disorders, while barium affects the circulatory system. Cadmium and chromium, for their part, enter the water from smelting and mining operations. Both affect the kidneys, and chromium also harms the liver.

  The lead in our drinking water merits special attention. This extremely toxic form of pollution affects a large portion of the population, often through the leaching of lead pipes or lead solder joints. About 10 million children—the most vulnerable among us—are exposed to large amounts of lead in their drinking water. Studies show that this toxic metal can impair the mental development of children and impede both mental and physical development in infants. Exposure to excessive levels also can result in central nervous system damage, kidney impairment, anemia and hearing loss.

In May 1993, the EPA released the results of its largest survey to date on lead poisoning in drinking water. The report found that 819 water systems, which together provide water to 30 million people, had excessive lead levels, according to a *New York Times* report. To conduct the EPA study, water systems were required to collect samples from certain houses in their territories and rank them by lead content. The content is excessive if the house in the 90th percentile—meaning only 10 percent had a worse lead level—contained more than 15 parts per billion of lead in its water. This federal standard was reduced from 50 parts per billion in 1992.[9]

Among water systems that serve more than 50,000 people, the houses with the highest lead contents were in the following cities: Charleston, South Carolina (165 ppb); Utica, New York (160 ppb); Newton, Massachusetts (123 ppb); Columbia, South Carolina (114 ppb); Medford, Massachusetts (113 ppb); Yonkers, New York (110 ppb); and Chicopee, Massachusetts (110 ppb). Ninety-two other houses, in 22 states and Washington, D.C., had anywhere from 16 ppb to 76 ppb.[10]

- *Fluoride.* A number of cities around the country have added fluoride to their drinking water, based on claims by the American Dental Association and the U.S. Public Health Service that the compound reduces tooth decay. In reality, no published studies prove this contention. But a variety of health disorders have been linked to fluoride, including skeletal damage, a condition called fluorosis (which makes teeth brittle) and cancer. According to one study comparing cities that fluoridate water with those that do not, this toxin accounts for 40,000 cancer deaths each year.

- *Mercury.* Like fluoride, mercury is a lethal pollutant deposited in our waters through industrial waste. This metal, used in paper, paint, vinyl chloride and fungicides, can damage the kidneys and the central nervous system. At high concentrations it is fatal. In one case in the 1950s, a Japanese factory dumped mercury salts into a bay and poisoned more than 100 people. Some suffered brain damage or went blind; 43 of them died. Closer to home, mercury from industrial dumping currently poisons many types of fish as it makes its way up the food chain. Mercury dumped in Washington and Oregon, for example, has been shown to travel about 2,000 miles and contaminates Alaskan seals.

Our Mounting Waste Problem

Considering the huge amount of harmful products we produce, it should come as no surprise that our garbage is a major health hazard. About 250 million tons of ignitable, toxic or corrosive waste is produced by American industry each year. Meanwhile, Americans produce about 200 millions tons of garbage a year, or more than four pounds a day per person.[11] The scope of the problem is enormous—toxic chemicals and nonbiodegradable plastics are buried in landfills, infectious waste from hospitals is dumped into sewage systems and then the ocean, and nuclear waste is contaminating our underground water supplies and soil.

The bulk of our solid waste is dumped into poorly lined landfills, from which health-threatening chemicals can leak into our water supplies. Other garbage is incinerated rather than dumped, but this process can emit a variety of toxins affecting our health and contributing to acid rain. To alleviate these problems, we must decrease our production of toxic waste and start serious efforts to recycle and compost garbage, both of which are viable alternatives to our current methods of waste disposal. The garbage crisis will only worsen until we take individual and collective action to get it under control. Today we face these problems with waste disposal:

Landfills. Most of our solid waste—some 80 percent—goes into landfills, which gained popularity over the years because they offered a "cheap and easy" way to dispose of trash. The short-sighted reasoning seemed to be, "Let's not worry about how much waste we produce or how toxic it is. We'll just dump it in the ground and forget about it." But the price tag attached to this disposal method conveniently excludes the cost of cleaning up leaks and providing health care to people who are harmed by the sites' toxic contents. And while our reliance on landfills as a mode of disposal has declined in the past decade, the primary reason is that many are becoming filled to capacity.

The toxic substances in landfills pose a tremendous threat to our health. In fact, a General Accounting Office study from the early 1980s reported that some 378,000 dump sites across the country may be a serious health threat. The study found that a toxic-waste dump of one sort or another was contained in every county of every state. The toxic contents of these sites can be hazardous for centuries, giving them plenty of time to leak through the linings of the dumps and contaminate underground waterways and the surface environment. That's if the toxic-waste dump has a lining. One EPA survey found that many treatment and storage sites do not.

Despite the prevalence of toxic dumps, many Americans simply do not know where the sites are located and, therefore, may never consider that a dump in their community is having adverse effects on their health. Yet the evidence shows that people living near toxic dumps have much to worry about. One study, conducted by New Jersey's University of Medicine and Dentistry, suggests that hazardous waste disposal is one of the biggest problems we will face in the coming years. This study tracked the mortality rates in 20 cities and townships in northeastern New Jersey. It found a strong correlation between the presence of toxic waste sites and cancer deaths. Indeed, the death rate for various cancers—stomach, esophagus, larynx, lung and colon—was 50 percent higher than the national average in areas having a high concentration of hazardous dumps.

The New Jersey study showed us the connection between toxic disposal sites and cancer rates in one small area of the country. But consider that in the 1980s the EPA developed a priority list of 850 sites posing a threat to the public health while the Office of Technology Assessment (OTA), for its part, identified 10,000 priority toxic-waste sites for clean-up. The government's ability to clean up these sites is highly questionable, especially in light of the results of the Superfund program of the 1980s.

The $1.6 billion Superfund program, under the direction of the EPA, was supposed to clean up thousands of leaking dumps, but only six sites had actually been tended to—in a slipshod manner, at that—when the program ended in 1985. Later, Superfund became a scandal when it was found that the EPA had negotiated with major polluters to relieve them of future liability and perjured itself before Congress. One-third of the money that supposedly was spent on cleanup activities could not be accounted for by Congress.

Incinerators. These so-called "resource recovery systems" got their start in the 1970s and now number more than 180. This method of disposal uses huge furnaces, kilns and boilers to turn hazardous waste into massive amounts of ash. While incinerators are promoted as a pain-free solution to our toxic-waste problem (by burning the waste, we avoid the tougher and more necessary step of reducing the amount we produce) they are proving to be quite harmful to the environment and our health.

According to the consumer group Stop Incinerators Now, incinerators emit both furans and dioxin, the carcinogenic substance found in Agent Orange. They also emit health-threatening gases such as nitrous oxide, hydrochloric acid and sulfur oxides. All three of these gases contribute to acid rain, and nitrous oxides also are a primary offender in ozone depletion. Other toxins released by the furnaces, such as the metals arsenic, lead and cadmium, have been correlated with cancer and neurological disorders. The incinerator ash itself is then disposed of in landfills, adding to the existing problems with toxic-waste sites.

In May 1993, the Clinton Administration took some action to get the pollution caused by incinerators under control. According to a May 18, 1993 report in the *New York Times*, Carol Browner, head of the EPA, called for an 18-month freeze on the development of new hazardous-waste incinerators. The freeze was targeted primarily at 164 incinerators nationwide that burn about three million tons of hazardous waste each year. The new program also stated that incinerator owners must apply for permanent operating licenses and scientifically assess the health and environmental risks posed by their facilities. And, finally, the federal government will set new levels for the amount of dioxin and heavy metals incinerators can emit into the environment.[12,13]

In calling for the freeze, said the *Times*, a hazardous-waste specialist at the EPA wrote a memorandum outlining "numerous flaws in the government's program for overseeing cement kilns and industrial furnaces." Among these flaws: Many incinerators do not have trained personnel, many do not comply with air-pollution requirements at the federal and state levels, and many types of chemical waste are fed into furnaces without a thorough analysis of their content. The end result is that tons of toxic chemicals can be released into the atmosphere by these incinerators. The EPA specialist was quoted in the *Times* as saying: "Since 90 percent of the liquid hazardous waste in this country and two-thirds of the sludge and solid hazardous waste are burned in cement kilns, the public is at significant risk."[14]

Nuclear Waste

In the 50 years since nuclear energy was first introduced during World War II, it has proven to be far from the "safe and clean" source of power promised by its promoters. The industry has a poor safety record, and research shows that power and weapons plants across the country have contaminated the water supply and soil with radioactive materials. These materials are released into the atmosphere and disposed of in dumps—some not even lined—where they will continue to pollute the environment for centuries to come.

In the coming years, the cost of cleaning up the radioactive and chemical pollution caused by this "inexpensive" source of energy will be steep indeed. The Department of Energy (DOE) estimated in 1989 that we would need to spend as much as $90 billion to clean up civilian and bomb-making plants under its jurisdiction, but that estimate was immediately challenged by some members of Congress, who believe the cleanup costs could climb as high as $200 billion. What's more, four DOE projects to "decommission" reactors, buildings and laboratories at nuclear sites across the country are expected to cost between $800 million and $1 billion each by the time they are completed, in some cases decades from now.

In the meantime, the materials processed in nuclear facilities—plutonium, uranium, strontium and other radioactive substances—are taking a tremendous toll on the environment. To take just one example, the Feed Materials Production Center in Fernald, Ohio, was found in early 1988 to have been releasing radioactive dust clouds into the air on a monthly basis due to faulty filters. Radioactive waste stored in leaking containers also was contaminating the area's groundwater. In late 1988, the government finally admitted—after many years of denial—that it had known for decades that the plant's normal operation would emit uranium and other substances. Even small amounts of radioactivity, it said, could be a health hazard to the people living in the Fernald area.

On the heels of that admission, a DOE report in late 1988 found that a number of nuclear weapons facilities were serious threats to human health. But with the help of the press, the government still claimed that while a threat existed, no harm had been done to anyone during decades of nuclear-weapon production, according to its "health surveys." These surveys, it turns out, resulted from computer simulations, not actual research of people living in the surrounding areas.

The reality is that radioactive and toxic chemicals, either singly or together, have damaged the environment at many nuclear facility sites across the country. In some sites, underground reservoirs used for drinking water or water used for irrigation has been contaminated; in others, toxic and cancer-causing substances are polluting the soil, groundwater and surface streams. The DOE's 1988 report cited such problems in the following locations:

- Lawrence Livermore National Laboratory, Livermore, California.
- Rocky Flats Plant, near Golden, Colorado.
- Pinellas Plant, Largo, Florida.
- Idaho National Engineering Laboratory, near Idaho Falls, Idaho.
- The Kansas City Plant, Kansas City, Missouri.
- Sandia National Laboratories, Albuquerque, New Mexico.
- Los Alamos National Laboratory, Los Alamos, New Mexico.
- Nevada Test Site, near Las Vegas, Nevada.
- Feed Materials Production Center, Fernald, Ohio.
- Portsmouth Uranium Enrichment Complex, Piketon, Ohio.
- Mound Facility, Miamisburg, Ohio.
- Savannah River Plant, near Aiken, South Carolina.
- Y-12 Plant, Oak Ridge, Tennessee.
- Pantex Facility, Amarillo, Texas.
- The Hanford Reservation, near Richland, Washington.

Detoxifying Your Environment

Considering the magnitude of our pollution problems, it's not surprising that many people don't know where to start in seeking solutions. But, as always, the process of change begins with education and committed action. If you are interested in reducing the adverse effects of pollution, consider joining a group that supports such causes and subscribing to publications that will educate you about the issues.

Then, think about the actions you can take to detoxify your environment. To help solve the garbage crisis, for example, you can buy fewer nondisposable items and get actively involved in recycling and composting programs. To help stop the destruction of the Amazon forests—an environmental disaster driven in large part by our appetite for meat—you can choose to eat less beef. To reduce the amount of chemicals being poured down our drains, you can replace hazardous household cleansers with nontoxic substitutes, such as vinegar, borax, baking soda, natural oils and the like.

As for the chemical pollution in our environment, you can let manufacturers, retailers and politicians know you don't want harmful chemicals in consumer goods or harmful pesticides in your produce and other food items. You can choose to support companies and farmers who offer alternatives to such products. You can reduce your consumption of energy, heat and air-conditioning, and use your automobile less by opting for public transportation, car pooling, and walking and cycling when feasible. In the end, there's no shortage of ways to help reduce the amount of pollution in our environment and its adverse effects on everyone's health.[15]

II

The Poisoning
Of Our Food Supply

CHAPTER 2
Fertilizers

Ultimately, all forms of life depend upon plants, which are the only living organisms that can create life from inorganic matter. This process, called photosynthesis, allows plants to utilize the sun's energy to convert water, minerals from the earth and carbon dioxide from the air into carbohydrates, proteins and fats—the basic sources of energy for all living things. Science has not been able to recreate this deceptively simple chemical conversion in the laboratory. It can only devise ways to provide plants with nourishment, so that they may draw an even greater supply of food from the soil.

Ordinarily we think of soil as "dirt," something we walk on that is muddy in winter and dusty in summer. But soil is where nutrition begins. It contains the raw materials that provide us with shimmering fields of wheat, golden stalks of corn and plump strawberries. The topsoil, which serves as the growing medium for most plant foods, consists mainly of decaying rock particles and rock dust. The remainder, known as humus, is a mixture comprised primarily of decaying vegetable and animal wastes.

Inside this rich topsoil is a complicated world of living organisms that help plants assimilate minerals and chemical compounds from rock particles. Funguses, bacteria, earthworms and insects are among the many forms of life that feed on humus. These minute animals slowly decompose plants left from the previous growing season, as well as animal carcasses and manure. They also aerate the soil so that gases can be exchanged and water absorbed. As a result, sulfuric and carbonic acid are generated, which further the decay of rocks and release their mineral contents, thus enriching the soil.[1]

In the wild, nature maintains a constant ecological balance. Plants that have created life from the soil return to it in death, as do the animals that feed on plants. Absorbed and processed by the soil, the dead are recycled into the living. In nature there is no waste, no pollution.

Unfortunately, this perfect state no longer exists in the human food chain. Dramatic changes in our farming processes have destroyed the natural ecology of the soil, and most of this damage has been done in the past century by the use of chemical fertilizers, the overcultivation of the land and the practice of "monoculture," in which a few crops are overplanted.

For most of the 12,000 years since plants were first domesticated, farmers simply supplemented nature with organic fertilizers. They then rotated crops or let fields lie fallow so that the soil's nutrients would not be depleted. The earth was not made to produce more than it is constitutionally able to bear. The picture started to change in the early nineteenth century, when a renowned German chemist named Justus von Liebig discovered that plants could be artificially fertilized with chemicals. Von Liebig conducted a series of brilliant experiments to identify the chemical substances needed by plants. He burned numerous species of plants, analyzed the substances found in the ashes and determined that soil was merely a mixture of these substances. If humans were to provide these chemical substances, he believed, plants would obtain all the nutrients they needed.

As scientifically sound as this conclusion may appear, it failed to take into account that soil is more than its mineral content. Von Liebig all but ignored the organic, living components of soil that are contained in humus. As a laboratory chemist, he failed to understand that the varied network of underground life, from moles, mice and shrews to earthworms and microorganisms, is an indispensable, life-generating part of our soil. To von Liebig's way of thinking, all that plants needed were nitrogen, phosphorus and potash—and all of these could be artificially produced.

The Decline Of Our Soil

By the time von Liebig's artificial fertilizers were generally available, farmers in the United States had already robbed the land of one-fourth of its topsoil due to poor soil management.[2] The seriousness of the loss is readily apparent when we consider that it takes nature 500 to 1,000 years to replace a single inch of topsoil. Most of the early settlers and pioneers did not know how to conserve soil, and they did not or could not learn about it. After all, the land was free or cheap, and there seemed to be a never-ending supply of it. Their credo: "Get what crops you can out of the land; when it's burned out and can produce no more, move on."

The price of this random rape of the land was paid in the mid-1930s. Great dust storms formed over much of America's farmlands, blowing away clouds of black topsoil from recently plowed fields. The prairies had been overgrazed, trees that once broke fierce winds and held moisture in the land had been cut down years before, and the earth had dried out from overcultivation. Thousands of impoverished farmers were forced to leave their wasted farms and migrate to the still-fertile earth of California and the Pacific Northwest.

Today, farmers recognize the damage done to the soil by their ancestors, so they successfully combat the destruction of the soil wrought by wind and water erosion. But, at the same time, they have found a new way to destroy the land—by using chemical fertilizers to force it to produce more than it should. The process has been accelerated and amplified because the huge industrial farms of the agribusinesses industry have, for the most part, taken over the land of the small, conventional farmer who lived close to nature. Today, especially for those large farms, quantity is more important than quality in food production. The result: Most of America's farmlands have been polluted with artificial chemicals for the sake of profits.

Consequently, ecological balance no longer exists on most farms. The practice of monoculture—the overplanting of a few crops— has depleted the soil of certain essential trace elements. The self-contained environment of yesterday's farms has given way to a compartmentalized form of agriculture. Today's produce farmer buys meat from the butcher shop and milk from a store or dairy farm, instead of keeping cattle, chickens and pigs on the farm. In the process, he sacrifices animal wastes, a readily available source of natural fertilizer. This is an unfortunate loss, since soil dressed with manure produces crops that are more nourishing and better tasting than those grown in chemically fertilized soil. Chemical manufacturers perpetuate the myth that there is not enough organic fertilizer to go around, but the facts do not bear this out. In fact, animal waste in the United States amounts to billions of tons annually.[3] In other countries, manure is distributed to farms, an all-but-impossible task in the United States due to the concentration of our livestock breeding. Cows and pigs are contained in single feedlots that may hold as many as 50,000 animals and 250,000 chickens. It would be prohibitively expensive to collect and transport all that natural fertilizer to fields where it is needed, thousands of miles away.

In short, it is cheaper, cleaner and easier to transport bags of chemicals than tons of manure. But the end result is that our animal waste does not contribute to the food chain through the natural recycling process; instead, it is disposed of as sewage and pollutes the nation's water systems. In less than a century, humans have upset the balance of nature by robbing the soil of nutrients that are never returned to it. Even our waste is wasted.

Instead we use artificial fertilizers—nitrogen, phosphorus and potash (known to farmers as NPK)—which bring about changes in the composition of soil that destroy or seriously disturb the very organisms that benefit it. The presence of these organisms serves as a barometer of soil fertility. If they cannot survive, it is a sign that the soil will not bear crops worth eating. The work of earthworms and microorganisms is essential, but they are destroyed by these chemicals. Super-phosphate fertilizers tend to create acid conditions in which these organisms cannot survive. In Australia, for example, nine-foot-long earthworms originally present in vast numbers were completely exterminated by this type of fertilizer.

The reason artificial fertilizers destroy living things in soil is that their ingredients are highly water soluble. In nature, easily soluble fertilizing elements rarely occur. For example, the plant nutrients contained in humus dissolve in water very slowly, feeding plants at a rate that will not poison them and their living benefactors in the soil. In addition, proper fertilization involves more than applying three concentrated chemicals to the roots of plants. More than a dozen minerals and trace elements are needed as well. While these minerals and trace elements account for only one percent of a plant's needs, they are extremely important nutritional factors. Many human diseases result from diets deficient in these factors, which often are missing from foods grown in chemically treated ground.

Chemical fertilizer manufacturers were quick to respond when it was discovered that these elements were lacking in synthetic plant foods. They quickly mixed in a few, calling them such things as "power boosters," which did nothing to help the soil. All of these concoctions were totally imbalanced because they did not simulate the proportions that exist in nature. Consequently, the carbohydrate-protein ratio of many crops began to change for the worse, and vitamin content declined.

For an example of this phenomena, we need only look to the tomato. Once fragrant red orbs bursting with juice, tomatoes have become woolly, tasteless and tough fruits. Fertilizers and hybrid strains have been combined to produce tomatoes that have superior handling and keeping qualities. But what about the loss of vitamin C and flavor? Farmers, it seemed, had other problems to worry about. As their operations grew from patches and pounds to acres and tons, they realized that harvesting machines would damage normal, tasty tomatoes. So a pulpy, thick-skinned hybrid that could withstand rough handling was created.

What's more, the growing season for tomatoes has been unnaturally extended, because agribusinesses have created a year-round demand for fresh tomatoes. Grown during the winter in southern and western states, tomatoes cannot be left to ripen on the vine if they are to survive being shipped thousands of miles north. As soon as NPK forces them into existence, tomatoes are picked green and ripened artificially. During their long voyage in refrigerated trucks and trains, they are kept in temperature-and-humidity-controlled environments that effectively stop their growth. Just before they are sent to your local market, tomatoes are sprayed with ethylene gas, which turns them red. What the consumer gets is a nutritionally worthless, unripe, cosmetically treated product.

Excessive use of artificial fertilizers lessens the keeping qualities of many other food plants, making it necessary to pick them before they can absorb whatever nutrients are left in the soil and ripen naturally. Industrial farmers fondly point to the beautiful, uniform appearance of the produce as proof of the benefits of NPK. But consumers are forced to eat celery that is as pithy as it is pretty, melon-sized and mealy cucumbers, and strawberries big as plums but with less flavor than their cardboard containers.

The health of a plant is a complex matter that is not always reflected in its appearance. Crops regularly doped with chemicals never attain the optimum food value of their organic counterparts. The necessary trace minerals cannot be absorbed effectively, even when they are present in the soil, because in artificially fertilized plants, the beneficial effects of humus are thwarted, if not destroyed. It is the finely dissolved particles of humus that transfer most of the minerals from the soil to root hairs. Being negatively charged, humus particles attract positively charged minerals, such as potassium, sodium, calcium, manganese, magnesium, boron, aluminum, iron, copper and other metals. When nitrogen is poured into the soil year after year, both humus and root hairs become coated with it, and the transfer of minerals can no longer take place.[4]

Too much potash decreases the synthesis of ascorbic acid (vitamin C), carotene (vitamin A), chlorophyll and amino acids. Too much phosphorus produces a zinc deficiency in livestock and poultry, which are fattened on chemically produced grain. These animals pass these vitamin and mineral deficiencies on to us when we eat their meat. Humans, the last link in the food chain, inevitably suffer the consequences when man tampers with nature. Many medical researchers believe the relatively recent upsurge in degenerative diseases is directly related to the poor-quality foods produced by modern farming methods.

The Green Revolution

Fifty years ago, the widespread use of chemical fertilizers and pesticides prompted the agricultural establishment to herald the arrival of a "green revolution." Super-hardy crops impervious to insect pests could now be grown in unending abundance, it was said, and the world's food shortages would soon end. By the early 1970s, the American farming industry was using nearly 45 million tons of NPK.[5]

Meanwhile, the protein content of farm crops began a steady downward slide. The promise of abundance was fulfilled, but at a big nutritional cost. Wheat yields per acre shot up dramatically when artificial fertilizers were introduced, for example, but the protein yield declined along the way. In 1940, Kansas wheat contained as much as 17 percent protein; that content fell to 14 percent in only 11 years, with the average yield being about 12 percent.[6] Starchy, cheap carbohydrates took the place of this life-giving foodstuff.

In essence, the "green revolution" tried to meet the challenge of world hunger with quantity, not quality. Chemical fertilizers weaken remaining proteins by upsetting the delicate balance of amino acids within their molecules. Their body-building, tissue-renewing qualities are seriously jeopardized. When a single amino acid is missing, as is often the case, the others refuse to do their job. If nonessential amino acids are not present, even though the others are, the essential ones may do only half their work. To meet its physical requirements, the body tries to compensate for these faulty foods by craving and eating more of them. But that hardly solves the problem. In the end, the practice of eating more and more protein foods, which the body can only partially utilize, wastes the very protein that is in short supply in terms of the world's needs and the most costly item in the diet.

We need to consider the real cost of manufacturing chemical substitutes for what the earth can produce more efficiently. For example, both cotton and nylon consist of long chains of small units of molecules linked together (monomers). The cotton plant takes the energy it needs to produce fiber from the sun and draws raw material from the soil. This process costs nothing and creates no pollution. Nylon, on the other hand, is made from petroleum—a fossil fuel consisting of stored plant energy of a millennia ago. To bind the molecules into monomers, petroleum or coal must be burned to power the machinery that spins out nylon.

Thus, great amounts of non-renewable energy sources are lost forever. The factory produces air pollution as a byproduct, and nylon and plastic gadgets, utensils, plates and cups litter the landscape forever. These chemical products are new to the life cycle and no microorganisms exist that can degrade and recycle them back to the soil. On a positive note, today's consumers can buy biodegradable products such as laundry and cleaning agents in their supermarkets and thereby help preserve the earth's ecology rather than destroy it.

Although the raw materials of chemical fertilizers are abundant, the manufacturing process consumes an immense amount of fossil fuel energy. To that cost, add the price tag for transportation to farms and mechanical dispersal and you have a truer picture of the great waste that results from substituting the artificial for the real.

It also must be noted that modern farming methods—both the use of chemical fertilizers and the dumping of natural waste—pollute our waters. Untreated sewage eventually finds its way into

America's streams, rivers and lakes, along with disastrous amounts of NPK leached from the earth by irrigation and rain. Both can cause water plants to grow in abnormal numbers and sizes, which then use up the oxygen dissolved in the water. This process kills fish and other water animals that depend upon oxygen for life and takes away the water's self-purifying ability. Dissolved oxygen can change small amounts of pollutants, including industrial wastes, into harmless substances. But massive amounts of fertilizer have overwhelmed nature's defenses, and many bodies of water have become foul and practically lifeless.

As the August Institute of Ecology reported more than 20 years ago: "It is a gigantic one-way flow of elements from the earth and the air into the sea. The scale of the operation is far greater than anything previously known on the face of the earth. And this human phenomenon is in stark contrast with the natural communities of plants and animals which have been living in balance with their surrounds for thousands of years."[7]

This one-way flow of essential elements can be stopped if a concentrated effort is made to feed back the nutrients we now rob from nature. Organic fertilizers must be substituted for artificial ones; waste products must be processed and recycled if the closed system in which we live is to survive.

The Effects Of Nitrogen

The prime component of chemical fertilizers is nitrogen (nitrates) produced in the laboratory. Runoff water containing nitrates often seeps into farm ponds and wells, rendering them unfit for human and animal use. Cattle that drink nitrate-contaminated water lose weight and can no longer utilize their feed completely. Cows show the symptoms of nitrate poisoning by producing less milk, and what they do produce is of inferior quality. If not treated at once, the animals soon die.

So do humans. Nitrogenous fertilizers have their most immediate and drastic effects on infants, who may be exposed to the chemicals through polluted water or vegetables that have absorbed a lot of fertilizer. Infants are susceptible to a disease called methemoglobinemia, which is caused by substances called nitrates. Nitrogen compounds can be converted into poisonous nitrites, a similar substance, by certain bacteria in the stomach. When nitrites enter the bloodstream, they react with hemoglobin (the red pigment in the blood) to form methemoglobin. Because hemoglobin carries oxygen to tissues and methemoglobin does not, the victim may turn blue and, in some cases, suffocate and die. While the stomachs of infants contain less acid than do those of adults, their intestinal flora contain certain types of bacteria that facilitate the transformation of nitrate to nitrite.[8]

Scientific studies have shown that food and water can be dangerously contaminated by nitrates. In food, nitrates saturated in soil tend to accumulate in the leaves and stems of certain plants, especially spinach, beets and carrots. Canners of these vegetables are plagued by the problem of internal corrosion of the cans due to excessive levels of nitrates. Twenty years ago, a study at the Missouri Agricultural Experiment Station also found that several brands of canned baby food contained as much as 40 milligrams per two-ounce jar. This amount was well in excess of the 12 milligrams of nitrogen as nitrate recommended as a maximum daily consumption limit for infants by the Public Health Service.

Another problem with having high levels of nitrates in both drinking water and produce is the nitrates' ability to induce cancer-causing substances known as nitrosamines. Researchers have noted the high incidence of stomach cancer in Japan, Chile and Iceland, where large quantities of fish are eaten. These fish contain high levels of nitrates due to the leaching of chemical fertilizers into the waters. (Other factors that may contribute to the rate of stomach cancer are the high content of polyunsaturated fat in fish and traditional habits of eating rapidly.) For Americans, nitrosamines are more of a problem due to their indiscriminate use as a preservative for such foods as luncheon meats, salami, hot dogs, ground beef, ham, bologna and frankfurters. But more about that fact later.

Other Agricultural Tricks

In addition to using chemical fertilizers to produce an abundance of nutritionally inferior food, agribusinesses apply other chemicals to crops to alter both their growth process and their appearance on supermarket shelves. One group of chemicals is used to "suspend" the growth of crops so that farmers can pick them at their leisure, rather than waiting until they have reached their peak of flavor and nutrition. Treated this way, supermarket produce looks fresher than it really is. But the fact that these chemicals can stop or delay the life-processes of a living organism is cause for alarm. The question is, can these growth inhibitors also arrest human growth? Until that question can be answered beyond a doubt, these chemicals should be banned.

Still other chemicals are poured over plants to increase their size. Americans are particularly proud of the size of their produce, and agricultural fairs give prizes to the biggest cabbages, melons and tomatoes, even though they are not the best. Inside, treated vegetables and fruits tend to be mealy and tasteless, having used up the nutrients they were designed to produce in their own struggle for outrageous growth.

Our "fresh" produce gets another round of assault from artificial dyes—such as those used on the rinds of some oranges—and from the waxes and mineral oil used to coat pears, apples, plums and other fruits to make them look more attractive and improve their keeping qualities. The FDA approved the direct application of these substances on fruit and vegetables in 1964, after years of permitting only their packaging to be coated. That such waxes were also used to polish floors seemed to cause little concern among the guardians of the nation's health. Germany banned such coating in 1938.

Finally, much of this produce is sprayed with a toxic group of chemicals known as phenols to preserve them during their long journey to the marketplace. Even in doses as small as 1.5 grams, phenols are so lethal that they can induce vomiting, circulatory collapse, convulsions and decay of the mouth and intestinal tract if swallowed. The FDA originally stipulated that produce treated with phenols be identified by a sign, but that requirement was discarded under pressure from agribusinesses. In Germany and Italy, phenol-treated American citrus fruit must be stamped with the words: "With Diphenyl. Peel Unsuitable for Consumption."

Back To Nature?

The widespread use of chemicals to grow the raw abundance of nature is truly disheartening. As long as we rely on artificial fertilization, it is only a matter of time until all our soil is made useless for growing crops. Ecologists worry that a time may come when there is no more land to cultivate. It has been estimated that the total destruction of fertile soil and the accompanying disappearance of all plant life on earth would mean the extinction of all animal life within one year. This frightening fact may best express how dependent humans and other animals are on the proper and natural use of soil.

There is no way to circumvent the life cycles of the soil for long. They are intrinsic, essential and far-reaching. We can disrupt them, but we cannot prevent the ensuing devastation that will inevitably result. Only through organic agriculture—working with natural materials that are the core of soil structure—can we cooperate with nature in an intelligent and fruitful manner. It is time for us to realize that we are only one small part of the food chain. We can never control it, but we can destroy it and ourselves in the process.

CHAPTER 3
Pesticides

Every day, about 860 people in the United States suffer from pesticide poisoning. That's 315,000 poisonings a year from chemical substances contaminating our air, soil, water and food supply. The worldwide death rate from pesticide poisonings tops 200,000 a year, but agribusiness has defended the use of these toxins on the grounds that they protect crops from the ravages of pests, fungi and weeds. The reality is that the loss of U.S. crops due to insects has nearly doubled in the past 50 years, even though our use of insecticides has increased ten times over during that same time.[1]

What accounts for this seeming contradiction? For one, many pesticides are indiscriminate killers. They not only eliminate the insects, weeds and fungi for which they are intended, but also destroy the natural predators that eat other insects. By killing off predators such as mites, earthworms, centipedes and beetles, pesticides rob the environment of its natural checks and balances. And, in the process, they dangerously alter the ecological balance of the soil.

In addition, the widespread use of pesticides has led to the development of about 650 species of pests resistant to certain pesticides. Much like the bacteria that have mutated into new strains in response to our wide use of antibiotics, these super-resistant pests have outwitted mankind's technology by developing an immunity to our poisonous pesticide products.[23]

Many pesticides have health-threatening and carcinogenic properties. Pesticides such as the now-infamous DDT, as well as Captan, EDB and Alar, are highly toxic substances that pose the risk of cancer and other adverse health effects. But these poisons may be widely used for decades before we acknowledge their potency. DDT, for example, was used for 30 years before our government banned it in the early 1970s. And even though it has been off the market for two decades now, DDT continues to haunt us. Like other pesticides, it is stored in fat and becomes more concentrated as it moves up the food chain. In early 1993, a study showed that women with a high concentration of DDT residues were four times as likely to develop breast cancer than other women.[4]

Pesticides have become like an addictive substance in the agricultural industry worldwide. The more we use, the more dependent we seem to become on these harmful products. The United States is the world's largest user, accounting for one-third of all pesticide purchases. We spend a staggering $7 billion a year on these products, which include more than two billion pounds of active ingredients, with herbicides, fungicides and insecticides at the top of the list. A total of 21,000 pesticide products are available for use in the United States.[5] Although agriculture accounts for the lion's share of pesticide use, we also apply these products to our lawns, parks and golfing courses and in our homes, schools and factories.

Not surprisingly, substances so widely used become pervasive in the environment. They are carried across the land by wind and rain, and infiltrate the air, soil and water. One pesticide, methyl bromide, has even been linked to the destruction of the earth's protective ozone layer. Thirty years ago, Rachel Carson detailed the devastating effects of this widespread contamination in her revolutionary book, *Silent Spring*. She showed that the poisons in pesticides threaten whole species of birds, fish and animals with extinction due to reproductive failure. Some of the species include bald eagles, hawks, blackbirds, quail, pheasants, falcons, foxes and raccoons.

In a weird twist on pesticide toxicity, farmers in 40 states have claimed that a product produced by E.I. DuPont killed the very crops it was intended to protect. This product, called Benlate DF, was introduced in the 1970s to combat fungi in crops. But after the company launched a new powdered version of Benlate DF in 1987, it began to have problems with contamination in the manufacturing process. DuPont took the product off the market in 1991 and paid a whopping $500,000 million in damages to farmers who claimed the product had destroyed their crops. Then it refused to pay any more. In an ongoing court case, a federal district judge said DuPont managers had withheld information about the disaster and fined the company $1 million.[6]

The residues of pesticides also lodge in the foods we eat, such as grains, fruits and vegetables, meat and poultry and even canned goods that roll off mass-production lines. According to the EPA, these residues pose more of a threat to public health than air pollution or hazardous-waste dumps. In addition, the groundwater in at least 38 states is now contaminated by pesticides. More than half of the U.S. population relies on this groundwater as a source of drinking water, according to estimates by the EPA. Concentrations of various pesticides, such as DDT, PCBs, heptachlor and chlordane, have been shown to store in the tissues of various animals, as well as in human fat tissue and even mothers' milk.

A study conducted in the early 1980s in rural farm areas of Quebec, Canada, points out the potential dangers of widespread pesticide use. The study examined the link between agricultural pesticides and mortality rates in the region for three types of cancer—cancer of the brain, lymphatic tissues and leukemia. After categorizing 34 drainage basins according to low, intermediate or high pesticide sales, the researchers found a correlation between several pesticide-use variables and cancer deaths, with varying links depending on the gender and age of the subjects. Generally, men had an excessive rate of leukemia, while women had a high incidence of lymphatic-tissue cancer.[7,8]

Agricultural workers, of course, are at particular risk for the adverse effects of pesticides. Studies have linked occupational pesticide exposure to an increased risk of diseases such as leukemia, brain glioma, Parkinson's Disease, lymphoma, soft-tissue sarcoma and tumors of the skin, prostate and stomach.[9,10] One study conducted in Iowa and Minnesota, for example, found a significantly increased risk of leukemia for farmers exposed to the insecticides used on animals.[11] In recent years, researchers have called for a closer examination of the effects of chronic pesticide exposure on the nervous system of workers. Because the very purpose of some pesticides is to act on neural tissue, the neurotoxicity of these chemicals requires more extensive testing than they have received to date.[12,13,14]

Regulating Poisons

Despite the potential risks, pesticides that are known to be dangerous—or about which we know very little—continue to be used. A decade ago, the EPA said that more than 200 pesticides on the market had not been proven safe through valid scientific testing. Today, about 90 pesticides have been identified as known or potential carcinogens by the EPA. Fifteen of the particularly hazardous pesticides in worldwide use today were identified in Rachel Carson's *Silent Spring* in the early 1960s.

The FDA and the EPA, which are responsible for regulating our pesticides, have established so-called "tolerance levels" for these substances, or the amount that can be tolerated without adverse health effects. These levels are established by first determining the point at which there are "no observable effects" in laboratory animals, such as nervous-system impairment and cancer. That figure is divided by 100 to arrive at a more sensitive tolerance level for humans.

But this process is not only arbitrary in determining human sensitivity, but also based on incomplete data. In 1984, the National Academy of Sciences estimated that only 10 percent of the pesticides in use had sufficient data to conduct a full evaluation of their health hazards. The potential risk for serious health effects—including birth defects, genetic damage and cancer—has not been studied in many pesticides.[15]

Indeed, pesticide tolerance levels may have little relation to their actual safety. C.K. Winter of the University of California's Department of Food Science and Technology has reported that the allowable levels of pesticides in the diet may pose more than the "negligible" health risks permitted by our federal standards. Writing in a scientific journal, Winter states: "The common and logical views that 'legal' residues are 'safe' while 'illegal' residues are 'unsafe' are not supported by scientific evidence." He believes the tolerance levels are useful as legal-enforcement and international-trade tools, but that they do little to benefit the public health.[16]

The EPA has attempted to relax our safety standards for pesticides in recent years. In 1988, it began to permit "negligible levels" of cancer-causing pesticides to be used in processed foods. While the Delaney Clause of the Food, Drug and Cosmetics Act (1958) bans the use of such pesticides in processed foods, the EPA took the stance that pesticide residues in such foods were not covered by the clause. On this basis, the agency deemed one case of cancer for each one million people to be an acceptable risk. However, the National Academy of Sciences has determined that, according to this guideline, the potential cancer risk for just 28 pesticides would be nearly 1.5 million cases over the course of 70 years, or 20,700 cases a year.[17]

In mid-1992, a federal court disagreed with the EPA's interpretation of the Delaney Clause, and told the agency that the residues of cancer-causing pesticides could not be permitted in our processed foods. But Carol Browner, the new head of the EPA under President Clinton, has given signals that she will uphold the agency's position on permitting the use of such pesticides. In early 1993, she said the 35-year-old Delaney Clause was outdated and that the pesticides it keeps off the market do not pose "an unreasonable risk to public health," as reported in the *NYCAP News* published by the New York Coalition for Alternatives to Pesticides, Albany.[18]

At the same time, it is ironic that a 1992 audit of the EPA's pesticide-labeling procedures by the agency's Office of the Inspector General, found that toxicity studies supporting many pesticides were old, incomplete and in general disarray. Of 95 pesticides reviewed in the audit, toxicity studies could not be located for more than one-third, according to *NYCAP News*. Beyond that, 58 pesticides did not have full sets of studies available and may not do so until the EPA's reregistration of pesticides is finalized in 2002. In addition, the audit found that some products had obsolete toxicity studies older than the EPA itself. Finally, half of the pesticides' labels did not adequately state precautions about use, and the EPA's files did not contain final printed labels for 24 of the pesticides.[19]

The Poisons In Pesticides

There are two primary types of pesticides—organic chlorines and organic phosphates. Here's how a few of these chemicals contaminate the environment and pose a threat to our health:

DDT. In April 1993, researchers at Mount Sinai Medical Center in New York released the results of a breast cancer study. They concluded that women with the highest levels of DDT residue in their blood had four times the risk of developing breast cancer as women in a control group. In fact, the control subjects had 35 percent less DDE (the residue substance of DDT) in their blood than the breast-cancer patients. This study established the clearest connection to date between DDT, an insecticide long recognized as toxic, and breast cancer.[20]

The study also demonstrated one of the truly dangerous aspects of rampant pesticide use: Though DDT was banned for most uses in 1972, the deadly chemical was identified as a culprit in cancer 20 years later. That's because DDT, a widely used organochlorine compound in the decades leading up to its ban, can remain intact as it works its way up the food chain. It then accumulates in the fat tissues of animals and humans, particularly the kidneys and liver, from where it can inhibit body functioning. In fact, DDT can retain half of its toxicity for more than a decade, and one study has shown that for every one unit of DDT in the blood, there are more than 300 units in fat tissue.

The irony is that DDT was thought of as a "miracle" chemical in the 1950s—one that would liberate us from diseased insects and thereby reduce the incidence of diseases such as malaria and typhus. Eventually, though, as billions of pounds of the substance were used in the United States, it became clear that the toxin was lethal to various types of birds. That's when researchers discovered how DDT could travel through water, dust, resistant insects and the food chain itself, endangering even human life in a variety of ways. The question, as always, is why we allow such products on the market when we know dangerously little about their properties and potential effects on health?

Heptachlor and chlordane. These two insecticides also belong to the organochlorine family of chemicals. They were introduced in the 1940s and widely used for three decades before we restricted their use because of their cancer-causing properties.

Both chemicals were used on a wide variety of plants. In addition, they were sold for residential use on lawns and golf courses. While other countries began to restrict the use of these insecticides as early as the late 1950s, the United States waited another two decades before it acknowledged their harmful effects: The use of chlordane was limited in 1975; three years later, we stopped the use of heptachlor for everything but termite control.

Like DDT, chlordane and heptachlor lodge in fat tissue. Chlordane has been linked to stomach cancer, in particular, and a 1987 study by the EPA found that it poses a high cancer risk when used as a termite insecticide in homes. In the late 1980s, heptachlor's use in seed grains continued to pose a cancer risk. In one case, hundreds of thousands of chickens were found to be tainted with this persistent pesticide and had to be destroyed. In another case, contaminated milk produced on dairy farms in three states had to be recalled because it contained high levels of the carcinogenic substance.

Polychlorinated biphenyls (PCBs). As with DDE (the residue of DDT), PCBs have been linked to breast cancer. In a study conducted in a hospital in Hartford, Conn., the level of PCBs and DDE in women with malignant breast tumors was 50 to 60 percent higher than in control subjects. Indeed, the average PCB level in the cancer biopsies was about a thousand times higher than the level deemed to be safe in food by the FDA.[21]

Another problem is that the fat-soluble PCBs can be transferred to infants through breast milk. In 1991, a German study showed that the concentration of PCBs in breast milk was three to five times higher than the level permitted in cow's milk. The researchers found that the fat tissue of more than 260 infants and children had seriously high concentrations of organohalogens.[22]

Dieldrin, endrin and aldrin. The United States began to control the use of these three organochlorines in 1976—and with good reason. Studies have shown that all three are damaging to animals, causing central nervous system damage, cancer and birth defects. Aldrin, for example, forms a substance called dieldrin once it is in the body. This potent substance stores in fat tissues and poisons both the nervous system and the brain. Aldrin also has been shown to cause sterilization and reproductive problems in rats and quail. Endrin, for its part, forms three new harmful compounds in the body.

Methyl bromide. This 60-year-old insecticide is one of the ten most commonly used in the United States. More than 40 million pounds are used here each year to fumigate soil before planting takes place. The pesticide also is used in food factories and warehouses, as well as on a variety of food commodities, including produce, cheese, pasta and baby foods. Methyl bromide exposure has been associated with birth defects, and it may be carcinogenic in humans. It also affects the central nervous system, causing symptoms such as speech disorders, loss of muscle control and depression. Severe poisonings can be fatal.

In recent years, methyl bromide has been identified as a primary culprit in the destruction of the ozone layer. Since this layer protects us from the sun's ultraviolet radiation, its depletion is expected to increase the rate of skin cancer and cataracts and to weaken our immune functioning. Methyl bromide releases free radicals in the stratosphere. Free radicals, the primary cause of aging and disease, are unpaired electrons that cause cell damage by attacking fatty acids and causing lipid peroxidation. They are far more potent than the chlorine released by chlorofluorocarbons (CFCs), the chemicals responsible for much of the destruction of the ozone layer.[23]

2,4-D, 2,4,5-T and dioxin. All three of these herbicides were ingredients in Agent Orange, the chemical defoliant used in Vietnam. Dioxin, in particular, is an extremely lethal chemical, but the other two also are highly toxic.

In 1992, the National Cancer Institute reported that the widespread use of these phenoxyacetic herbicides, and especially 2,4-D, has been linked to significant increases in the incidence of non-Hodgkin's lymphoma (NHL). The report said the rate of NHL has increased by more than 50 percent since 1977. In Kansas, Nebraska, Canada and Sweden, studies show that the use of 2,4-D is related to a two- to eight-times rise in the incidence of NHL. The use of 2,4-D and other lawn pesticides by dog owners also has been linked to malignant lymphoma in dogs.

The study concluded: "Since the use of pesticides, particularly phenoxy herbicides, has increased dramatically preceding and during the time period in which the incidence of NHL has increased, they could have contributed to the rising incidence of NHL."[24]

Parathion and aldicarb. These two insecticides are organic phosphates, and their properties are similar to those of lethal nerve gases. They destroy certain enzymes in the body that are needed to protect the nervous system from a chemical transmitter that impairs its functioning. Parathion is so lethal that it causes hundred of deaths each year. It has been used on a wide variety of crops, including fruits, vegetables, grains, tobacco and cotton, and its residues have been shown to last for as long as 16 years.

Aldicarb, also known as Temik, is a highly popular agricultural pesticide. Insects develop deadly disorders of the nervous system when they eat a plant treated with Temik. Not surprisingly, then, laboratory tests also have noted a link between low-level exposure to Temik and neurological disorders, miscarriages and cancer. Large doses of Temik have caused convulsions, muscle spasms and death in humans. In 1985, 2,000 people in Bhopal, India were killed when one of Temik's base chemicals leaked from a Union Carbide plant.

Ethylene dibromide (EDB). This pesticide, in use since 1948, has the greatest cancer-causing ability of any chemical, according to the National Audubon Society. While most of the EDB we produce is used as an additive in gasoline, tens of millions of pounds are used each year to kill root worms and to fumigate fruits, vegetables and grains in storage. In the 1980s, one EPA survey found that nearly 60 percent of grains had detectable amounts of the chemical, and an FDA survey found that nearly all harvested fruits contained the residues of EDB.

Alachlor. More than 80 million pounds of alachlor are used each year, making it one of our most widely applied herbicides. In the mid-1980s, laboratory tests linked alachlor, which goes by the trade name of Lasso, to cancer, and the EPA began a study to determine whether alachlor should be banned. Three years later, the agency stated that the alachlor contained in our waters was indeed a "cause for concern." Nonetheless, the EPA decided to leave alachlor on the market because its cancer-causing risk fit within the agency's definition of a "negligible" risk.

In addition to the products described above, the litany of harmful pesticides includes many others. Among them are the following: chlordimeform (CDF), dibromochloropropane (DBCP), lindane (BHC), hexachlorocyclohexane (HCH), pentachlorophenol (PCP), paraquat and camphechlor.

The Organic Solution

Can we produce the foods we need without the use of pesticides? Though the agriculture and chemical industries would have you believe otherwise, the answer most certainly is "yes." We did it before the use of pesticides soared in the 1950s, and many organic farmers are doing it today with great success. Remember that our growing dependence on pesticides does not stem from a true need for the products, but rather from the chemicals' ability to destroy natural predators and create resistant insect strains. We are caught in a vicious cycle, with more and more pesticides required even as our crop losses continue to mount.

Organic farmers are committed to producing foods without the use of fertilizers, synthetic pesticides, naturally derived toxic pesticides, additives and preservatives. They also rotate crops to nourish the soil and maintain its ecological balance, in contrast to conventional farmers who often rob the soil of its nutrients by planting the same crop year after year. Some of the natural pest-management methods used by organic farmers include beneficial insects that control various other pests, and a harmless, nontoxic bacteria (in a spray form) that kills mosquitos and black flies.

While organic foods currently cost consumers a bit more than conventionally produced foods, the success of today's organic farmers undoubtedly will draw others into the industry. As more farms practice organic methods, efficiencies will be achieved and in turn retail prices should decrease.

By supporting organic farmers, you can go a long way toward avoiding pesticide exposure and letting the food industry know that you don't want a mouthful of poisons with every bite you take. It's also a good idea to support the development of diversified food-growing systems in your local community and region, and to grow some of your own fruits and vegetables when possible.

In the end, a safe food supply doesn't seem like too much to ask for. But the EPA has shown that it will allow harmful pesticides on the market, based on its analysis of the relationship between a pesticide's cancer-causing risk and the "economic benefits" of its use, such as lower food prices. That line of reasoning merely results in "tolerance levels" and "negligible-risk levels" for dangerous synthetic pesticides. Surely we can do better in the regulation of these products, given their impact on our air, water, soil and food supplies.

CHAPTER 4
Food Additives

Just about all the food we eat is chemically treated at each stage of the production process. By the time it reaches the supermarket shelf, our food has been processed to the point that it has little in common with its original state. All commercially processed foods, whether of animal or plant origin, have their growth pattern, size, appearance, texture and nutritional value manipulated and transformed by an array of chemicals, many of which may be hazardous to our health. Here, we will look at the various chemicals added to food during the final stage of production, when they are processed and packaged.

These chemicals, which fall into the general category of food additives, range from reasonably benign food colorings to highly dangerous preservatives such as sodium nitrate and sodium nitrite, which contribute to the formation of cancer-causing toxins in our bodies. Depending on the food in question, it may have been treated with degerming agents, chemical flavorings, synthetic dyes for coloring, flavor enhancers, stabilizers, mold inhibitors, aging agents, preservatives, bleaches, emulsifiers, conditioners, and so on.

Plainly put, we are eating fake and adulterated food that has been stripped of much of its nutritional value. The problem is not just what we are eating, but what we are not eating as well. Denatured foods are highly processed and laden with chemicals. They do not contain the natural nutrients that are needed to sustain good health. For instance, processed cheese may be a combination of water, vegetable oil, powdered casein and milk protein. Breads and cereals may contain BHA or BHT, calcium propionate, glycerides, conditioners and emulsifiers. And the foods sold as "substitutes"—such as margarine, bacon bits, artificial whipped cream and nondairy creamers—are filled with chemicals, colorings, preservatives and saturated fats.

More than 2,900 food additives are now in use. The FDA, whose job it is to ensure the safety of our food supply, maintains a database of detailed toxicological information on nearly 1,700 regulated direct food additives; an additional 1,200 direct additives are included in the database, but the data on them are less extensive. While this may sound reassuring, the reality is that the safety of any food additive is never guaranteed. When the FDA deems a chemical additive to be "safe," it is assuring us with a "reasonable certainty" that the substance will not be harmful when used as intended. The permitted level of an additive in food is called the acceptable daily intake (ADI). This approach was established in 1961 by the Joint Food and Agriculture Organization (FAO)/World Health Organization (WHO) Expert Committee on Food Additives.[1,2]

Given the vast number of additives, discussing all of them would be impossible. In the pages that follow, we'll look at a sampling of food additives that may pose a threat to human health.

BHT And BHA

BHT (butylated hydroxytoluene) and BHA (butylated hydroxyanisole) are petroleum products used in foods and other items. They were first designed as fat stabilizers that would replace the natural oxidants lost when refined fats and oils are processed. But the safety of these additives has never been demonstrated, and some experiments have suggested that they have toxic effects on cells. One recent experiment measured the cytotoxicity of BHT and BHA on several types of cultured human cells. For all of the cell types analyzed, BHT was more cytotoxic than BHA.[3]

Over the years, BHT and BHA have been used in many processed foods, including lard, chicken fat, butter, cream, shortening, bacon, potato chips, processed meat and fish, pastries, cakes, candies, peanut butter, nutmeats, raisins, milk, imitation fruit drinks and breakfast cereals. BHT and BHA are used in the containers for milk, ice cream, cottage cheese, cereals, potato chips and cookies. Finally, they are added to chewing gum, drugs and cosmetics.

One would assume that any substance in such wide use had undergone conclusive safety tests. But this is not the case. At least one of the studies on which the approval of BHT was based, for example, was financed by three BHT manufacturers and produced conflicting results. In this 1955 study, four species of animals were fed various amounts of BHT. Researchers determined what single-dosage amount would kill the animals, and what lower level the animals could tolerate over a two-year period. Some animals on the lower dosage died, but their deaths appeared to be unrelated to the BHT. Some of the control animals, which did not receive BHT, also died. Based on this limited evidence, the researchers concluded that BHT had not caused any of the deaths.

In the 1950s, experiments conducted in Romania revealed that rats fed BHT experienced metabolic stress. Eventually the Romanian Hygiene and Public Health Institute recommended that BHT be banned from use in foods. And in 1959, Australian researchers found that BHT in lard reduced the growth rate and weight of male rats. The reduced growth rate was directly attributable to BHT. They also found that BHT led to an increase in liver weight, perhaps due to the extra stress placed on the organ, which is responsible for the detoxification of toxic substances.

However, researchers at the Cleveland Clinic reported in 1972 on a possible connection between the use of antioxidants and a decline in the number of deaths from stomach cancer. Antioxidants, substances such as vitamins C, A, E, zinc and selenium, pair with cell-damaging free radicals' unpaired electrons and therefore neutralize their destructive capacities. The researchers pointed out that stomach cancer was the leading cause of cancer death among men in the United States in 1930; by 1970, it was the fifth-leading cause. Their reasoning: Breakfast cereals, which contain some natural antioxidants, began to be widely used in the United States in the early 1930s. And in the late 1940s, when chemical antioxidants came into use, the decline of stomach cancer accelerated. Yet a similar fall in the stomach cancer rate did not occur in Europe, where breakfast cereals were less popular.

People who are sensitive or allergic to BHT and BHA have experienced reactions such as skin blisters, hemorrhaging of the eye, weakness, edema and breathing discomfort. But in this age of chemical additives, it is difficult to detect the cause of an allergic reaction, and equally hard to determine what chemicals a product contains. The label on a product containing BHT or BHA may merely list a "freshness preserver" or "antioxidant." Such "information" is of little use to those who want to avoid these chemicals.

Sodium Nitrite And Sodium Nitrate

These additives are used extensively in cured meats and smoked fish. In fact, a quick survey of the packaged meat shelf of any local supermarket will show you just how many products contain sodium nitrite. Nitrites are used most often (although nitrates were used originally); nitrate itself is not actually a curing agent, but serves as a source of nitrite.

The toxic factor in nitrates from vegetables, especially spinach, can cause a relatively rare disease called methemoglobinemia, to which infants are particularly susceptible. When this condition occurs, the blood's hemoglobin, which carries oxygen to the body tissues, is changed into methemoglobin. Because methemoglobin is unable to transport oxygen, the person turns blue and becomes dizzy. In extreme cases, death may result.

The link between sodium nitrite and cancer is what worries scientists and consumer advocates. Nitrite participates in a chemical reaction that results in a particularly potent cancer-causing substance. Here's what happens: When nitrite combines with certain amines in a mildly acidic environment, such as the human stomach, it forms nitrous acid. The nitrous acid then reacts with the amines to form nitrosamines, which are among the most potent carcinogens yet discovered by scientists. (Amines result from protein breakdown and are found in some drugs and other nonfood substances; only the amines called secondary and tertiary react with nitrite to form nitrosamines.)

One of the most alarming characteristics of nitrosamines is that they do not limit their attack to one body organ, such as the lung or stomach; instead, they appear to be able to produce cancer in any or all parts of the body simultaneously. What's more, no species of animals has been found to be resistant to them. They have produced cancer in hamsters, mice, rats, dogs, guinea pigs and monkeys. There is no reason to think that the human species is exempt.

Nitrosamines were first discovered to be cancer-producing in

1956 by British scientists. In 1963, a German chemist put forth the idea that nitrosamines might be produced in the stomach by a chemical reaction involving nitrite. Some 80 percent of the nitrosamines used in animal studies have proved to be carcinogenic. Some have produced cancer at extremely low dosages, or even after a single dose. Other times, nitrosamines given to female animals toward the end of pregnancy left the mother unaffected, but caused the offspring to later develop cancer of the liver, kidney, brain and spinal cord.

Unfortunately, the human stomach appears to be an ideal environment for the production of nitrosamines. A nitrosamine called diethylnitrosamine was produced in the stomachs of cats and rabbits fed as little as two hundred parts per million of nitrite—the amount allowed in meat and fish—along with the amine diethylamine. This result is especially significant because the stomachs of these animals are of approximately the same acidity as the human stomach. The acidity level, in turn, has some impact on the rate of nitrosamine formation.

In one series of experiments, Dr. William Lijinsky of the Oak Ridge National Laboratory in Tennessee, fed nitrites and amines to test animals, which developed the same kind of cancer as animals who received the corresponding nitrosamine. These studies yield virtually indisputable proof that the dangerous nitrosamines can be produced in the stomach when nitrite and amines are consumed. In one of Dr. Lijinsky's studies, a group of rats were fed nitrite and an amine found in a particular drug. Within six months, 100 percent of the rats had developed malignant tumors. A substance is considered to be a potent carcinogen if it produces cancer in 50 percent of a group of test animals.

There seems to be little question that when nitrite and amines are present in the stomach at the same time, nitrosamines can form—and that most of these nitrosamines may be highly carcinogenic. Obviously, we can't change the fact that our stomach is an ideal acidic environment for nitrosamine formation. Nitrosamine-producing amines, too, are relatively difficult to avoid. They are found in wine, beer, tea, cereals, fish, cigarette smoke and numerous drugs, including anesthetics, tranquilizers, diuretics, antihistamines, antidepressants, oral contraceptives and high-blood pressure medications.

Nitrite should be the easiest to avoid of the three factors needed to form nitrosamines. Small amounts in some water supplies and certain vegetables are difficult to avoid, but most of the nitrites we ingest are those added needlessly—they are used only for cosmetic purposes—to meat and fish. In fact, another problem is that nitrosamines can form in the meat itself. The FDA and USDA have found nitrosamines in various types of processed meat, including dried beef, cured pork, ham, hot dogs, bacon, smoked chub and salmon. Some of these meat products contained anywhere from 11 to 80 parts per billion; some brands of bacon had more than 100 parts per billion after cooking.

With such evidence against nitrites, one might wonder why their use continues to be permitted. It seems that the FDA was influenced by various economic pressures to approve the use of a chemical it once classified as a harmful substance, according to "The FDA and Nitrite," a report written by Dale Hattis. Incidentally, Hattis was only able to obtain FDA documents concerning its approval of the use of nitrite in smoked fish after filing a Freedom-of-Information suit in 1972. He reported that, in 1948, the FDA stated in an information letter: "We regard [nitrite and nitrate] as poisonous and deleterious substances not required in the manufacture of any food subject to the jurisdiction of the Food, Drug and Cosmetic Act, and, as such, any food subject to the act and containing any quantity of these chemicals would be deemed to be adulterated, under the law, regardless of labeling."

But many members of the meat industry and government had an answer to that position. They claimed that nitrites were needed to protect against botulism, an often fatal form of food poisoning caused by a bacterium. The USDA held nitrites would damage the spores (reproductive cells) of the bacteria during cooking. Thus, if the bacteria later break out of their spores, they cannot grow or reproduce. However, the amount of nitrite permitted in meat far exceeds the level that would be needed to control botulism were botulism really the main concern.

The FDA began to allow manufacturers to use nitrite and nitrate for cosmetic purposes in 1960—as a color fixative in smoked tuna, smoked and cured salmon, shad and sable fish. Then, in 1963, several people died from botulism after eating smoked whitefish that had not been properly processed. This tragedy gave the fish industry an excuse to request permission for further use of nitrites. But despite this stated purpose for using nitrites, the FDA admitted in a 1970 report on the chemistry and toxicology of nitrites that sodium nitrite is used primarily as a color fixative—not a way to prevent botulism—in meat and fish.

Food Colorings

More than 90 percent of the colorings used by food manufacturers are synthetic, and most are coal-tar derivatives. Food colorings are added to nearly every kind of food and beverage found in the supermarket, including meats, soft drinks, wines, bread, cakes, cereal and fruit. By using these dyes, manufacturers can make a food the color they think consumers associate with quality—and thereby create the illusion of quality. For instance: They can make fruits and vegetables appear to be fresh off the vine—which they most certainly are not; they can make meat look fresh and juicy; and they can make other stale foods look appetizing.

Many consumers think the term "U.S. certified artificial color" means the safety of a coloring is assured. But of 19 dyes certified by the FDA in 1938 under the Food, Drug and Cosmetic Act, nine had to be "decertified" 20 years later when laboratory tests found them to be carcinogens. Some of the food colorings that have been delisted are Sudan I; Butter Yellow; Yellow #1, #3 and #4; Red #32; Orange #1 and #2; and Red #1 and #4. The safety of other dyes, including Red #3, Citrus Red #2, Red #40 and Yellow #5, also has been called into question. And the FDA banned Red #2 in 1976 because of its cancer-causing properties.

There is no justifiable reason for the use of artificial dyes in food—even those that have so far proven to be safe. The long-range effects of many food additives are not yet known. A two-year study of tartrazine (Yellow #5) found that the dye was not carcinogenic in mice.[4] But in a plant experiment, this dye and four others—Orange B, fast green FCF, indigo carmine and metanil yellow (a non-permitted dye)—caused a significant increase in polyploid breaks and micronucleus formation. High doses caused chromosome aberrations.[5] In a double-blind test, tartrazine and benzoates (another food additive) affected the central nervous system of two children, causing headaches, overactivity, learning difficulties and depression.[6] As for Yellow #6, there is some indication that it may affect the eye when ingested in large quantities.

Coal tar dyes. When heated in the absence of air, coal is converted into coke, coal gas and coal tar, which is a viscous black liquid. About 95 percent of the synthetic colorings used in the United States are coal tar derivatives. Red #2 is the most infamous of these, but the safety of other coal tar dyes also has been debated over the years.

The history of Red #2 shows us just how far the FDA and the

food industry will go before relinquishing a hazardous substance. Until banned in 1976, Red #2—known as amaranth—was used alone or with other dyes to color a vast range of foods. Products that have contained this dye include ice cream, ice milk, luncheon meats, frankfurters, processed cheese, fish fillets, cornflakes, shredded wheat, rolls, pretzels, cookies, cake mixes, pickles, fruit juice, canned fruit, salad dressings, jam, candy bars and soft drinks. Red #2 also was used in lipstick, other cosmetics and various drugs, including vitamins prescribed for pregnant women.

Red #2 was suspected of causing cancer as far back as 1956, but the debate heated up in 1970 when the FDA received translations of two Russian studies on Red #2. One study showed that extremely small amounts of the dye caused birth defects, stillbirths, fetal deaths and sterility in rats. Rat fetuses were endangered by only 15 milligrams of dye per kilogram of body weight—the same amount set by the World Health Organization as safe for human consumption. All in all, the evidence was strong that the dye was linked with both cancer and reproductive damage.

But the FDA claimed that there was no cause for worry and that Red #2 was above suspicion. The agency dismissed the Russian studies as invalid on the grounds that none of the animals in the control group had developed tumors; normally some cancer is found in control animals as they age. However, one of the FDA tests used as evidence of the dye's safety, conducted in the 1950s, was later found to have several serious inconsistencies, including a mix-up in which rats had been fed the coloring.

Under public pressure, the FDA announced in late 1971 it would severely lower the permitted level of Red #2 beginning in 1972. This would constitute a ban, in effect, since the amount allowed would be too low to be of any use to the food industry. But the food industry pressured the FDA to get an objective opinion from a group such as the National Academy of Sciences. The committee established by this group came to the conclusion that it was unnecessary and premature to restrict the use of Red #2, but its report was widely criticized for its obvious bias in the interpretation of scientific evidence. Red #2 was finally banned in 1976, six years after the FDA knew of the Russian studies and two decades after it was first suspected of being a carcinogen.

Other dyes. The safety of other dyes also has been questioned over the years. Historically the litany of questionably safe dyes have included Violet #1, which has been shown to cause skin lesions and malignant tumors in rats. This dye is used to stamp the USDA inspection symbol on meat and to color beverages, candies and pet foods. Likewise, tests have indicated that Citrus Red #2 may be carcinogenic. Florida growers have used this coloring to cover up the green skins of oranges, primarily in the fall season. A number of states banned the sale of artificially colored oranges after the FAO/WHO Expert Committee on Food Additives recommended in 1969 that Citrus Red #2 not be used on foods.

There also is question about the safety of Orange B, whose chemical structure is similar to that of Red #2. This dye is used mainly to coat frankfurters. A 1988 study of mice found Orange G to be both clastogenic and genotoxic, with chromosome aberrations occurring at a minimum dose of 25 mgs. per kilogram of body weight.[7] Red #3, for its part, was identified as a potentially carcinogenic dye by a Congressional committee in 1985. It is used by maraschino cherry makers, drug makers and cosmetics manufacturers. Large amounts of Red #4, also used in maraschino cherries, may lead to atrophying of part of the adrenal cortex and changes in the bladder.

Finally, it bears mentioning that Caramel Colour III has been shown to depress the immune system in mice, especially those whose diet is low in vitamin B6. In feeding studies, this color additive decreased the number of white cells and lymphocytes in the mice.[8] On the other hand, a human study of elderly males with a marginal vitamin B6 deficiency found that the acceptable daily intake of Caramel Colour III—when ingested for seven days—did not affect any of the immune factors investigated. Caramel Color III is used in beers and a variety of foods, including some types of sauces, gravies, soups, vinegars and bakery goods.[9]

Other Food Additives

In addition to the highly questionable food additives—such as sodium nitrite, BHT and BHA, and certain dyes—thousands of other additives find their way into our food. Many additives have proven so far to be nontoxic, while others are being studied for potentially negative health effects. What follows is a brief look at some of the additives listed frequently on food packages. The better you understand what you are eating, the more you can gain some control over the amount of pollution in your body.

Artificial flavorings. Two-thirds of the food additives used in the

United States are either natural or synthetic flavorings. These flavorings enable the manufacturer to skimp on the more expensive, genuine ingredients. Regulations governing flavorings tend to be lenient, in part because the flavors are generally used in very small amounts. That's no guarantee, of course, that a flavoring will not be hazardous to our health. Safrole, which was used as a flavoring in root beer until 1960, was found to cause cancer of the liver.

Food companies are allowed to declare that a chemical is "generally recognized as safe" (GRAS). Although flavorings are not actually classified as GRAS, they are handled in a similar manner: a manufacturer can declare a flavoring safe on the basis of very little testing. The manufacturer does not even have to list flavorings specifically on the label. Practically anything could be listed as an "artificial flavoring."

Benzaldehyde (benzoic aldehyde). This essential oil may be derived from almonds or produced synthetically. It occurs naturally in almonds, cassia bark, bitter oil, cajeput oil, tea, raspberries and cherries. It is used in apricot, brandy, rum, peach, liquor, cherry, berry, butter, coconut, pistachio, almond, pecan, vanilla and spice flavorings. It is also used in ice cream, candy, ices, beverages, cordials, baked goods and chewing gum. It may cause a skin rash and is narcotic in high concentrations. Large amounts produce convulsions and central nervous system depression. The fatal dose is approximately two ounces. This substance is on the GRAS list.

Benzoyl peroxide. This chemical is used to bleach flour and often is combined with aging agents, such as azodicarbonamide, iodate and bromate. Most of it decomposes to benzoic acid, which has been shown to have negative effects on the skin (urticaria and angioneurotic edema) and respiratory tract (asthma and rhinitis) in allergic or sensitive people.[10,11] Benzoyl peroxide also destroys vitamin E, which is important to know if one insists on eating products made from bleached flour.

Brominated vegetable oil. Commonly called BVO, this additive consists of vegetable oil combined with bromine. Flavoring oils are added to BVO, and the solution is then added to fruit-flavored drinks, both carbonated and noncarbonated. The bromine, which increases the density of the oils, keeps them dispersed throughout the drink so that they will not float to the top.

Manufacturers are not required to list BVO on labels. Yet tests have shown that rats fed BVO suffered damage of the heart, liver, thyroid, testicle and kidney. Studies conducted in England have found that fragments of BVO accumulate in animal tissue. Research must be done to determine whether BVO is able to cause cancer and/or reproductive damage.

Carrageenan chondrous extract (carrageenan). This is a glue-like derivative of Irish moss that has a salty taste. It is used as an emulsifier and stabilizer in chocolate products, chocolate milk, chocolate-flavored drinks, pressure-dispensed whipped cream, confections, syrups for frozen products, evaporated milk, cheese spreads, ice cream, sherbets, frozen custard, ices, French dressing and artificially sweetened jellies and jams. Ammonium, calcium, sodium and potassium salts of carrageenan are used in syrups, jellies, puddings, baked goods and beverages. Medicinal syrups also use carrageenan to sooth mucous membrane irritation. Sodium carrageenan has been on the FDA's list for study of mutagenic, teratogenic, reproductive and subacute effects, but is on the GRAS list.

Diethyl pyrocarbonate. DEPC is a chemical that prevents the growth of microbes in fruit drinks and alcoholic beverages. It has been used more widely in Europe than in the United States. Unfortunately, DEPC has been found to combine with ammonia to form a potent carcinogen called urethan. DEPC is never listed on labels because the chemical itself breaks down before the drink reaches the consumer. However, this fact does not rule out the presence of small amounts of urethan.

Disodium phosphate. A sequestering agent used in evaporated milk, macaroni and noodle products. It is used as an emulsifier in cheeses. It has USDA clearance for use in preventing cook-out juices in cured pork shoulders and loins, cured, canned and chopped hams and bacon. Disodium phosphate is also used as a buffer in adjusting acidity of chocolate products, beverages, enriched farina and sauces and toppings. Medicinally, it has uses as a cathartic, purgative and to treat a phosphorus deficiency. It can irritate the skin and mucous membranes. This substance is on the GRAS list.

EDTA. EDTA is used to prevent fat and oil products from becoming rancid. Foods such as salad dressings, oleomargarine, sandwich spreads and mayonnaise contain it. EDTA also is used to prevent processed fruits and vegetables from turning brown. It works by trapping impurities in the food. In fact, physicians treat metal poisoning with EDTA injections. When present in excessive amounts, EDTA can cause kidney damage, calcium imbalance and a condition resembling a vitamin deficiency.

Glycerides. This family of emulsifying and defoaming agents includes monoglycerides, diglycerides and monosodium glycerides of edible fats and oils. They are used in bread and other baked goods to maintain softness (by absorbing moisture from the air), and in ice cream, ice milk, milk, beverages, shortenings, lard, oleomargarine, chewing gum, confections, chocolate, sweet chocolate, whipped toppings and rendered animal fats. Diglycerides have been on the FDA list for study of possible mutagenic, teratogenic, subacute and reproductive effects, but are on the GRAS list.

Menthol. The menthol flavoring agent occurs naturally in mints, raspberries and betel nuts. The chief source of menthol is oil of peppermint. It is used in caramel, fruit, butter, spearmint and peppermint flavorings in chewing gum, candy, ice cream, baked goods, liqueurs and beverages. Other uses include perfumes, cough drops, nasal inhalers and cigarettes. In large doses, it can cause severe abdominal pain, nausea, vomiting, vertigo and coma. The lethal dose in rats is 2.0 grams per gram of body weight. This substance is listed as GRAS.

Monosodium glutamate. This flavor enhancer, commonly known as MSG, is widely used around the world. The first indication that it posed any dangers came when Dr. Ho Man Kwok discovered what he called the "Chinese Restaurant Syndrome." After eating in a Chinese restaurant, Dr. Kwok experienced headaches, tightness in his chest and burning sensations in his forearms and at the back of his neck. The cause was finally traced to the MSG, especially the large amounts used in soups.

In 1969, Dr. John Olney of the Washington University School of Medicine in St. Louis, found that large amounts of MSG fed to infant mice destroyed nerve cells of the hypothalamus—the area of the brain that controls the appetite and other important bodily functions. MSG also has been found to damage the retina of infant rats and mice, but the human eye, being more developed at birth, is less susceptible to such damage.

Research also suggests that MSG reactions may be related to the development of late-onset bronchospasm, which can occur up to 14 hours after food has been eaten. Pregnant women should restrict their intake of MSG, since some scientists question whether large amounts could have adverse effects on fetuses.[12,13]

Propyl gallate. This antioxidant often is used with BHT and BHA. In a 1965 study, researchers found that high levels of propyl gallate caused damage to the mitotic (cell division) mechanism of the liver cells. Further and more extensive research is indicated, especially because this is a widely used additive.

Salts. One study in Japan examined the effect of various salts— including sodium salts, potassium salts, a calcium salt and an ammonium salt—on the stomach of mice. The results suggested that the salts of food additives may promote the development of tumors in the glandular stomach mucosa of mice.[14] In addition, an epidemiological study in China established a link between the development of nasopharyngeal carcinoma (NPC) in children and preserved and salted foods. According to the study of 128 mothers of children with NCP and 174 controls, there was a significant link between the risk of NCP and the intake of salted fish, salted duck eggs, salted mustard greens and chung choi (a type of salted root) during weaning.[15]

Sodium citrate. This odorless additive, which comes in the form of crystals, powder or granules, has a salty taste. It prevents "cream plug," the semisolid collection of fatty material at the top of a container of cream, and "feathering" when cream is added to coffee. Sodium citrate is used as an emulsifier in evaporated milk, ice cream and processed cheese; as a buffer to control acidity and prevent loss of carbonation in soft drinks; and is also used in fruit drinks, confections, jams, jellies and preserves. This additive is on the GRAS list.

Sorbitol. Sorbitol is a white, crystalline powder with a sweet taste. It is found in berries, cherries, plums, pears, apples and seaweed, where it occurs due to the breakdown of dextrose. Sorbitol is used as a sugar substitute for diabetics, but its safety for this use has not been proved. It also is used as a sequestrant in vegetable oils, a thickener in candy, a stabilizer and sweetener in frozen desserts used in special diets, and a humectant (retainer of moisture) and texturizing agent in soft drinks, shredded coconut and dietetic fruits. The FDA has asked for further study of sorbitol.

Sulfiting agents. These additives, including sulfur dioxide and sodium and potassium salts of sulfite, bisulfite and metabisulfite, have been the culprit in many adverse food reactions in the past 10 years, generally among people who are asthmatic. By the late 1980s, in fact, sulfiting agents—along with aspartame, an artificial sweetener—had generated the largest volume of consumer reports to the FDA's Adverse Reaction Monitoring System. The food, beverage and pharmaceutical industries use these sulfiting agents as preservatives and antioxidants.[16]

The effect of sulfites on asthmatic people has been the focus of a number of studies. In one study, seven patients with asthma or rhinitis experienced severe or even life-threatening reactions when they consumed wine, salads and other foods treated with sulfites.[17] In a double-blind challenge of five sulfite-sensitive people with asthma, two had severe reactions to sulfite-treated lettuce. The reaction was life-threatening for one of the patients; the other had a severe reaction even though the lettuce contained only 30 percent of the usual sulfite dose.[18]

According to another study, however, the likelihood of a negative reaction to sulfite depends on the food in question, the amount of residual sulfite in the food and the patient's sensitivity. In this study of eight asthmatic people, four or less had negative reactions to various sulfited foods (such as lettuce, dried apricots and white grape juice).[19] However, it goes without saying that asthmatic people must take care to avoid these potentially harmful additives, both in store-bought products and in restaurants.

For those who are interested in a comprehensive look at food additives, we suggest *A Consumer's Dictionary of Food Additives* by Ruth Winter (Crown Publishers, New York) and Beatrice Trim Hunter's *Food Additives and Your Health* (Keats Publishing, New Canaan, Conn.). These two works list thousands of additives and describe them in detail.[20]

CHAPTER 5
Irradiated Food

As if the chemicals in our food were not enough to worry about, the U.S. government supports the addition of another harmful step to the food-making process. This one not only poses a potential threat to our health, but also sounds like weird science: The Department of Energy (DOE), responsible for disposing of our vast stockpiles of nuclear by-products, has proposed that we expose food to radiation. And the FDA has approved the "food irradiation" process, as it is called, based on what opponents say is slim and faulty evidence that the resulting food products will be safe for human consumption.

To the American public, which has become increasingly wise to the dangers of food-processing methods, it seems unlikely that we would even entertain the notion of irradiating food. Nonetheless, food irradiation surfaced as a serious proposal in the 1980s, when the DOE was looking for ways to recycle our high-level nuclear waste, including radioactive substances such as cesium-137, cobalt-60, strontium-90 and plutonium-238.

As one can imagine, developing disposal methods for such waste is no simple mandate. These substances are the legacy of a 30-year nuclear build-up, and they now present an enormous disposal problem. Nuclear waste facilities across the country are awaiting deactivation, and some estimates put the cost of "decommissioning" these Cold War relics at hundreds of billions of dollars. Meanwhile, no one wants such waste dumped in his or her own neighborhood, so the government had to come up with another way to handle the problem.

With that in mind, in 1985 the DOE established its Advanced Radiation Technology Program, originally called the By-Products Utilization Program, to research alternative methods of putting radioactive waste to use. Food irradiation, first explored in the 1950s as a way to preserve food for the U.S. Army, was an obvious target. After all, food is an absolute essential; if this huge market were to incorporate irradiation in its production process, it would create a tremendous demand for the nuclear industry's recycled waste. To promote irradiation, the government focused on two selling points: The process would not only extend the shelf life of foods, but would also kill harmful bacteria transmitted to humans via the food supply.

Today, the food-irradiation concept is beginning to pick up steam. A Florida company, Vindicator Inc., has established the first commercial irradiation plant in the country; a company in Utah has announced it will begin irradiating ground chicken breast to be sold in the Southeast; and the Department of Defense has stated it will buy millions of dollars worth of irradiated food for military use. What's more, irradiation's use as a food-safety measure has gotten a big boost from the rising rate of illness caused by foodborne pathogens, such as *Salmonella* and *E. coli* 0157:H7, the bacteria that caused several deaths and hundreds of illnesses in the Northwest in early 1993.

What Is Irradiation?

With this technique, food is exposed to ionizing radiation with either radioactive isotopes (cobalt-60 and cesium-137) or a large electron beam. In the process, the radiation kills bacteria and extends the food's shelf life significantly. Proponents of irradiation have likened the process to that of cooking, but clearly there are major differences between the two. For one, cooked foods become hot and tender; irradiated foods do not. And many foods approved for irradiation, such as fruits, vegetables and nuts, do not need to be cooked in the first place.

The cooking analogy is even more questionable given the chemical changes that take place in irradiated foods. Irradiation breaks apart the molecules of food, which then form new molecules and new chemicals when they come together again. The newly formed chemicals—called radiolytic products (RPs) and unique radiolytic products (URPs)—do not exist in any foods except those irradiated. With the microwave-cooking process, for example, food molecules are vibrated rather than taken apart; thus, no new chemicals are formed.

Scientists point out that RPs and URPs have not undergone rigorous testing on their toxicity. But the FDA has deemed the chemicals to be safe on the grounds that they are created in small amounts—specifically, 30 parts per million for RPs and 3 parts per million for URPs. That's far from a reassuring argument, considering that other substances have been shown to cause cancer in much smaller concentrations. The pesticide EDB, for example, causes cancer at just 3 parts per billion—1,000 times smaller than the level at which irradiation produces URPs.

In fact, opponents of irradiation have questioned the FDA's methods in granting the process a clean bill of health. When the FDA concluded that RPs and URPs are created in safe amounts, for example, it relied on a report put out by the Bureau of Foods' Irradiated Foods Committee. This report found that irradiated foods are "safe and wholesome" as long as the irradiation dose is smaller than 100K rad. As it turns out, however, the Bureau of Foods did not base its safety endorsement strictly on food experiments; it also incorporated some assumptions about the chemistry and physics of radiation.

These assumptions have worried some scientists. Irradiation is a far different process from cooking due to the huge amount of energy produced by ionizing radiation. This energy may alter the chemical make-up of foods in highly complex ways, perhaps increasing the level of carcinogenic or mutagenic substances already contained in foods or creating such substances for the first time. To assess the true cancer-causing potential of a process such as irradiation, it would have to undergo toxicological testing at large doses, said Dr. Richard Piccioni, a staff scientist at Accord Research and Educational Associates, in testimony before Congress.

The scientific validity of the studies used by the FDA to approve irradiation also has been called into question. Starting with more than 400 animal-feeding studies on irradiated food, the FDA eventually identified five that were both complete enough to warrant analysis and that concluded irradiated food is safe. But some of these studies lacked statistical significance and even indicated a potential health risk, as pointed out by Dr. Donald Lourie, chairman of the Department of Preventive Medicine and Community Health at New Jersey Medical School. In several studies, for example, rats fed irradiated foods experienced stillbirths and deaths for undetermined reasons.

More important, why was the FDA's approval based on so few studies, when thousands of experiments have been conducted over the past three decades on the effects of irradiation? Many of these studies have shown that irradiation has adverse effects on plants, animals and even children in one case. These effects include chromosome damage, autoimmune disease, a lowered sperm count and an increase in polyploid cells, one of the suspects in the development of leukemia. In a study of malnourished children in India, for instance, those who ate irradiated food developed these abnormal blood cells.

Also at issue is whether irradiation should be considered safe based on a short-term analysis of its effects. In China, the Ministry of Public Health set forth temporary standards for the irradiation of various foods after eight human trials found that the process had no effect on certain health parameters, such as weight, blood pressure, chromosomes and polyploidy. In these trials, 439 volunteers ate a diet for two to three months that included many irradiated foods, such as potatoes, rice, peanuts, mushrooms and sausages. But what does a three-month trial tell us about the potential effects over three years or three decades?

Despite these questions, proponents of irradiation have focused on the questionable benefits that might be derived from the process. They claim that irradiation offers a safe alternative to the use of pesticides and chemicals in foods, for example. But it's clear that the process would not eliminate the use of pesticides, which are applied to foods during the harvesting stage. Because irradiated foods are highly vulnerable to fungi and molds, they, too, would require post-harvest treatment with fungicides. In addition, it is not yet known if irradiation, like pesticides, will promote the development of bacterial strains that are resistant to the process.

A more likely benefit of irradiation, at least for food processors and grocers, is that it prevents foods from spoiling as quickly and extends their shelf life. The longer foods can sit on the shelf, the less the chance that supermarkets will lose money on items that spoil before they can be sold. But what about the consumer's viewpoint on this issue? To enhance the food industry's profits, we must eat food that has been unnaturally preserved. In fact, we could end up buying foods that appear to be quite fresh, but are actually stale.

Indeed, old foods have less nutritional value because their vitamin and mineral content deteriorates as they age. Irradiation will not prevent foods from losing their nutritional punch, but it will keep them looking "fresh" long enough that we end up eating them after the nutrients have been depleted. In fact, the very process of irradiation may destroy essential nutrients such as vitamins E, C and K, which would then have to be added back in to the products. This process of supplementation cannot duplicate the balance and mix of nutrients found in nature.

Why Ask Why?

Though proponents proclaim that irradiation is safe, one can only question the logic of subjecting our foods to more toxins. Many illnesses now plaguing the American public, including cancer and heart disease, have already been linked to the inadequacies of our modern diet. Our goal should be to consume more nutritious and fresh foods, such as fruits and vegetables, whole grains and legumes. Nonsensically, irradiation seems to point us in the opposite direction, since foods treated with radiation would appear to be fresh when, in reality, they are not.

Even so, the push for irradiation may be fueled by a growing problem in the food supply—the rising incidence of food poisoning from bacteria such as *E. Coli* 0157:H7 and *Salmonella*, contained primarily in animal foods. As also reported in *NYCAP News*, a March 1993 article in the *Wall Street Journal* stated that irradiation is "likely to become a big gun in the nation's food-safety arsenal." In fact, Mike Espy, the new Agriculture secretary under President Clinton, has stated that mandatory irradiation of all meat may be considered if livestock producers cannot get the pathogen problem under control. A study of irradiation's effects on the *E. coli* bacteria has been approved by the American Meat Institute, and Iowa State University is researching the process in relation to *Salmonella*, with financing from the U.S. Army.

In the meantime, a number of countries have banned the sale of irradiated food. These include Sweden, Germany, Australia and

Denmark. And while New York, New Jersey and Maine have imposed irradiation bans over the past few years, this legislation needs to be renewed at the federal level when the time-frame set by the ban runs out. If you oppose the process, take the time to get involved and let your representatives know what you think.

III

The Toxic Diet

CHAPTER 6

Sugar And Sugar Substitutes

Sugar is exactly as "pure" as the label on the bag proclaims. Its sparkling white crystals are clean and sterile, having had every trace of anything nutritious extracted from them in the refining process. Sugar has no vitamins, fats, minerals, proteins or any other nutrient essential to your health. The only thing sugar (sucrose) offers the body is quick energy from the calories it contains. It is an unadulterated chemical that has been linked to diabetes, dental caries, obesity—because it is composed largely of refined carbohydrates—and stomach problems.

But sugar tastes good. In fact, it is one of the most pleasant ways imaginable to gradually do yourself in. Sugar works its harmful ways very slowly, and the victim rarely becomes aware of the damage wrought until it is too late to reverse or even arrest it. The average American swallows about 150 pounds of sugar a year in any number of nutritionally inferior foods, thus making sugar a possible contributing factor to escalating illness rates.

The Empty Calorie

The typical American diet can easily contain 50 teaspoons of sugar per day, both prepackaged in foods and added at the table. These 50 teaspoons represent more than 800 calories, approximately one-third of the body's daily requirement of food energy. Pure carbohydrates such as refined sugar and flour seriously disrupt the body's metabolism because they provide cells with energy but do not feed them nutrients essential for their proper functions. Imagine that the human body is an automobile engine. If you were to put only gasoline (sugar) into the car and neglect to lubricate it with oil (vitamins, minerals, proteins and fats), the engine would soon break down. That process is what happens to your body when you displace nourishing foods like whole grains, cheese, raw vegetables and fruits with a chemical having no essential nutrients.

To utilize refined carbohydrates, the body must rob healthy cells of nutrients they need to survive. Indeed, the body leaches precious vitamins and minerals from itself in the process of digesting sugar, inducing a crisis state. Trying to restore an acid-alkaline balance to the blood, the metabolic system draws sodium, potassium and magnesium from various parts of the body, and calcium from the bones. So much calcium may be depleted that bones become brittle and vulnerable to fractures, while the teeth become susceptible to decay. Glutamic acid and other B vitamins are actually destroyed by the presence of sugar in the stomach, a condition evidenced in heavy sugar users by fuzzy thinking and a tendency to become sleepy during the day.

Often, as a result of eating sugar, the body does not have enough vitamins, minerals and proteins, such as enzymes, to complete the conversion of additional sugar into energy. Consequently, the carbohydrates are incompletely metabolized, leaving residues such as lactic acid. These poisons accumulate in the brain and throughout the nervous system, where they deprive cells of oxygen. Eventually, the cells die, making the body degenerate and become more susceptible to disease.[1]

Sugar manufacturers urge us to "eat sugar for quick energy," successfully luring nutritionally ignorant people into "sweet suicide." True, sugar does raise the blood sugar level temporarily, only to let it fall rapidly, even abruptly, a short time later. Sugar is absorbed into the bloodstream through the intestines within minutes of being ingested, producing a rush of "quick energy." But half an hour later the sugar is used up and a person is left with the familiar symptoms of hypoglycemia (low blood sugar): headache, dizziness, fatigue and irritability.

Studies show that refined sugar is actually a poor energy source. This research demonstrates that sucrose consumption lowers performance levels in children during play. Tests indicate that only 45 to 60 minutes after ingestion of sucrose, children suffer the most pronounced decrease in performance.[2] Still, their most common reaction is to reach for something sweet and repeat the process.

Since sugar in its natural state is a vital component of plants such as sugar cane and sugar beets, the raw material of sugar does contain valuable nutrients. The refining process, however, destroys all that is beneficial—eliminating some 24 food ingredients.[3] Potassium, magnesium, calcium, iron, manganese, phosphate and sulfate are among the discarded minerals; A, D and the B complex are some of the vitamins destroyed, and essential enzymes, amino acids, fibers and unsaturated fats are all removed. Most of the B complex vitamins are absorbed into a by-product known as blackstrap molasses, an excellent sweetener whose strong flavor generally prevents using too much of it. All the other important nutrients are in the residue which is processed as feed for livestock, who so far have shown no evidence of diabetes. So-called "raw" sugar is only white sugar to which a little molasses has been added for color and flavor, plus a few minerals, enabling the manufacturer to mendaciously label it "more nutritious."

Here's how the nutrients are lost: After the cane is harvested, it is chopped into small pieces which are crushed by huge rollers. Water is added and the juice is squeezed out, filtered and poured into heating vats. Powdered lime is then added to separate and coagulate most of the extraneous matter. The heated brownish liquid begins to clarify as the unwanted material settles to the bottom of the tanks. Moisture is boiled off until the liquid sugar is reduced to a thick, viscous mash, which is pumped into vacuum pans to further concentrate the juice. Nearly dry, the crystals are put into a centrifuge machine, where a residue of molasses is spun off. Again heated to the boiling point, the reliquified sugar is passed repeatedly through charcoal filters. Finally, it is condensed into crystals which are bleached. The resulting product is as pure a chemical as anything you might find in a chemist's laboratory.[4]

Noting that heart attacks, arteriosclerosis and strokes—common causes of death among diabetics—also became leading killers among non-diabetics in the twentieth century, famed British scientist Dr. T.L. Cleave identified sugar as the single common causal factor. He concluded that all these illnesses were actually different symptoms of the same "sugar disease," and that refined carbohydrates [such as white sugar and white flour] produced their harmful results in three ways:[5]

1. Refined sugar is eight times as concentrated as flour, and perhaps eight times as dangerous. The refined product deceives the tongue and the appetite, thus leading to overconsumption. Otherwise why would anyone eat 2½ pounds of sugar beets in one day? Of course, its equivalent in refined sugar is a mere 5 ounces. Overconsumption can lead to diabetes, obesity and coronary thrombosis, among other dangerous conditions.
2. The removal of natural vegetable fiber can produce tooth decay, gum disease, stomach problems, varicose veins, hemorrhoids and diverticular disease.
3. The removal of proteins can lead to peptic ulcers.[6]

As Dr. Cleave has pointed out, sugar consumption is only seconds old in terms of human evolution. The human desire for sweets was originally nature's way of tempting us to eat succulent and nourishing fruits and berries. These whole foods, coupled with natural grains, meats and vegetables, enabled humans to thrive and multiply through the ages. When civilized peoples were able to isolate the sweet-tasting chemical that had encouraged them to eat natural foods packed with vitamins, minerals and roughage, they disrupted the biological balance that had served them so well for so long. They then went on to combine refined sugar with adulterated, bleached white flour to produce entirely new and totally unnatural foods.

Because sugar is relatively inexpensive to produce, the food industry uses it as a filler to replace more expensive ingredients. It is unlikely that people would add as much sugar to the food they prepared as they readily accept in the "convenience" foods they buy. Manufacturers of cake mixes, for example, have found that the addition of copious amounts of sugar adds weight to the box and increases shelf life.[7]

Today, refined sugar is included in nearly everything we eat. By becoming increasingly more dependent on processed foods, we are ingesting more refined sugar than people did several decades ago, when three-quarters of all sugar consumed came from a bag bought at the grocery store. Today, only one-quarter of the sugar consumed is used at the table and for cooking. Besides the obvious processed foods such as cookies, cakes, desserts and soft drinks, sugar is listed as an ingredient in canned corned beef hash, ketchup, canned and powdered soups, salad dressings, peanut butter, boxed "hamburger-helper" dinners, cheese, TV dinners, luncheon meats and canned and frozen vegetables. Even sweet fruits are no longer considered palatable unless a thick syrup is added to the can or package. Moreover cigarettes, cigars and pipe tobacco contain sugar to satisfy this addiction. The only solution is to avoid all refined white sugar and bleached white flour in whatever forms they are disguised.

Artificial sweeteners are not a viable alternative, for they, too, cause degenerative disease. For example, cyclamate, an artificial sweetener derived from coal tar, was widely used in the 1960s until scientists discovered it caused bladder cancer and chromosome damage in laboratory tests. The FDA banned the poisonous substance in 1969, after it was on the market nearly 20 years. Moreover, these synthetic sweeteners keep alive a "sweet tooth," and it is only a matter of time before the user returns to sugar.

The best option is to choose desserts from the abundant, fragrant, juicy fruits of the earth. Pastries and cakes made from whole grain flours will reawaken tired tastebuds. Use these natural alternatives and sugar eventually will taste like the refined carbohydrate it is.

Blood Sugar Disorders

Hypoglycemia, or low blood sugar, has become a familiar complaint in our sugar-saturated age, but few have the knowledge or willpower to overcome it. When we eat, about 68 percent of all food, provided there is ample protein, is converted into glucose, a simple sugar similar to white sugar (sucrose), which supplies us with energy. The remaining 32 percent is used for repairing and building the body cells. The body can transform carbohydrates, fats and proteins into the type of sugar it needs to generate energy.

Low blood sugar can be reversed by replacing white sugar and flour with a diet rich in slow-burning proteins and natural carbohydrates, such as fruits and vegetables, plus a moderate amount of foods containing natural fats, such as soybean oil and avocados.

Refined sugars and starches, however, create havoc in the body's self-regulating mechanisms. Ordinarily, sugar is converted into glucose by the digestive juices and is carried through the bloodstream to the pancreas, which is stimulated into producing insulin. Excess sugar, in a more complex form known as glycogen, is stored in the liver for future use. When the blood sugar level begins to drop—a natural occurrence between meals—hormones signal the liver to convert some of its stored glycogen back into glucose. This reconstructed glucose is fed directly into the bloodstream, restoring a balance to the blood sugar level. In a properly functioning body, a healthy blood sugar level is maintained by the automatic interaction of insulin and hormones secreted by adrenal and pituitary glands.

Eating an excessive amount of sugar overstimulates the pancreas, which then produces an excess of insulin. Several things may happen. Most frequently, the person will develop an addiction to sweets to satisfy the insulin secretion. Or, the insulin will begin to convert too much glucose into glycogen and the blood sugar level will drop dangerously low, creating a condition that results in chronic hypoglycemia.

Diabetes, the opposite of hypoglycemia, results either from an inadequate supply of insulin and too much sugar in the blood or insulin not being properly used by the cells. Exhausted by the constant demand of producing insulin to convert all that sugar into heat and energy, the pancreas will finally malfunction and the excess sugar then pollutes the bloodstream. Without sufficient insulin to convert the sugar into glucose, the body is deprived of an essential food, and the diabetic remains hungry, no matter how much he eats. Sugar accumulates in the bloodstream faster than the body can excrete it through the kidneys in the urine, literally poisoning the victim. He becomes tired, weak and nauseated and can go into a diabetic coma, a condition causing death unless insulin is immediately administered.

Rather than instruct their diabetic patients to eliminate refined sugar, candy, soft drinks and other sweets from their diet, some within the medical establishment latched onto an imperfect alternative. After years of research, Canadian Doctor Frederick Banting discovered a way to extract insulin from animals in slaughter houses. In 1923 Dr. Banting received a Nobel Prize for his work. Drug companies, eager to exploit a captive market of a million or so diabetics,[8] a market that was destined to grow, pronounced Dr. Banting's work as one of the first "miracles" of modern medical science. As William Dufty pointed out in his valuable book, *Sugar Blues*, Dr. Banting later "tried to tell us that his discovery was merely a palliative, not a cure and that the way to prevent diabetes was to cut down on dangerous sugar bingeing."

"In the U.S. the incidence of diabetes has increased proportionately with the per capita consumption of sugar," Dr. Banting later wrote. "In the heating and recrystallization of the natural sugar cane, something is altered which leaves the refined products a dangerous foodstuff."[9]

Oral Problems

The consequence of indiscriminate sugar use is apparent in the deplorable condition of our teeth. Nearly all American adults are afflicted with tooth decay,[10] and the link between sugar and dental problems has been noted in other countries as well. In a study conducted by the Israeli Defense Forces from 1973 to 1986, for example, the unusually high incidence of dental treatments in armed service personnel was linked to the high per capita sugar consumption in their diet.[11]

Sugar feeds the bacteria normally present in the mouth, causing them to multiply. These bacteria adhere to the surfaces of the teeth, somewhat like barnacles adhering to the hull of a ship, and form a deposit known as plaque. Although tooth enamel is the strongest material in the body, the bacteria inside the plaque are able to eat through it and attack the dentine inside. A hole is eventually bored through to the pulp that feeds the tooth and the bacteria proceed to the root canal, causing a toothache and eventually destroying the tooth. Meanwhile, the excess sugar inside the stomach has depleted the body's calcium supply, further weakening the tooth's ability to protect itself.

The gums suffer equally because the soft, sticky nature of over-refined foods does not supply sufficient friction as the food is masticated to keep the gum margins hard, stimulated, and tight, up around the teeth. Pyorrhea (periodontal disease) is caused when plaque collects at the base of the teeth and forms into a hard deposit called tartar. Rather than affecting the teeth, the bacteria attack the gums and bones that support them. Bleeding and swollen gums are the first warning sign, and unless this difficult-to-cure disease can be checked, extraction of all the teeth will be inevitable.

The most effective way to eliminate tooth decay is to eat a proper diet. Since sugar is the main causative factor in dental caries,[12] they can be virtually eliminated if there is no sugar in the diet.[13] Studies further implicate sucrose as a primary culprit in the decreasing hardness of enamel; thus, it is the main source of cavities.[14] Many dentists also say that a good way to prevent tooth decay and gum disease is to eat a lot of chewy foods, such as apples. However, even the natural sugar found in fruit will encourage plaque formation, as will all carbohydrates. Brushing and flossing, therefore, remain all-important.

Coronary Disease

For years, doctors, scientists and nutritionists believed that an excessive intake of saturated fats, such as milk, butter and cheese, was a primary contributing factor to heart and artery diseases, two leading causes of death in this country. It has long been known that certain people, especially those who are overweight, develop a fatty deposit known as cholesterol on the inside of arterial walls. Over time, the cholesterol deposits clog the arteries, hardening and narrowing them until the blood cannot pass freely to the heart. Circulation is impaired and the heart receives an insufficient supply of oxygen. The person tires easily and develops leg cramps and chest pain. The artery may close off completely, causing a massive heart attack.

Dr. Cleave was the first to offer evidence that animal fats are not the only culprits in this process; sugars are guilty as well. Research indicates that diets rich in sucrose and fructose increase the metabolic risk factors associated with heart disease.[15] After all, the fats contained in eggs, cheese, butter, milk and meat were a staple of our diet long before debilitating circulatory diseases became an epidemic in Western countries. While we unwisely consume large amounts of these animal fats, their proportions do not near those of refined carbohydrates. When we fail to produce sufficient insulin to convert sugar to glucose, the result is a high blood sugar level and an increase in a blood lipid (fat) known as triglycerides. Evidence suggests that the triglycerides do the greater part of the damage to circulatory tissue.

In conducting his research on sugar, Dr. Cleave studied African tribes whose members live near urban, westernized peoples. In primitive tribes, diabetes and coronary disease were practically unknown, while relatives who went to the cities to work—and consequently started eating large amounts of sugar—soon began to show the familiar symptoms of deterioration. "Of one thing the author is very confident. The key to causation of coronary thrombosis lies in the causation of diabetes (and also of obesity)," stated Dr. Cleave in his important book, *The Saccharine Disease*.

Other Negative Effects

With each person consuming about 3½ ounces of cane and beet sugars a day, the effects of sugar on health has become a major medical concern. Although experimental data give strong indications that dietary sugar and easily absorbable carbohydrates are not directly responsible for the development of diseases, high sugar consumption combined with a reduction of other nutritive sources may be.[16] Here are some problems linked to sugar consumption:

Obesity. Surplus sugar is stored by the body as fat. When the liver has all the glycogen it can absorb, the excess glycogen is spilled into the bloodstream in the form of fatty acids. Transported throughout the body, these liquid fats are deposited in least-exercised areas such as the buttocks, stomach, thighs and breasts. When these areas can absorb no more, the fat is stored in major organs such as the kidneys and heart, causing a decrease in their functioning and eventual physical deterioration. The end result is that tissues throughout the body may be severely damaged.

Obesity is directly related to overconsumption of refined carbohydrates, and, because of the addictive nature of sugar, excessive food consumption is more likely with carbohydrate-rich diets. Although the fat content in food has experimentally shown to be the most important factor in obesity,[17] sugar, through its high energy density, may indirectly lead to obesity and diabetes as well as to early arteriosclerosis.[18]

Gastrointestinal disorders. Roughage is conspicuously absent from the diets of Americans and other industrialized Western peoples. Vegetable, fruit, grain and bean fibers are necessary for cleaning the teeth and massaging the gums while we eat. Inside the intestines, the fibers expand with water to produce soft, easy-to-pass stools. Moving through the intestines, these vital fibers also act as a natural cleansing agent, removing any bits of debris that might cling to the intestinal walls. Constant ingestion of over-refined foods like sugar and white flour leads to hard, compacted stools that are difficult to evacuate, resulting in constipation. The problem of body pollution is then further compounded by adding an irritating laxative chemical to the intestinal tract.

Straining to eliminate dense, sluggish waste matter from the bowel can cause colitis (an infection or obstruction of the colon), or diverticulosis (a pouch in the wall of an intestine), which may then become infected. Continued irritation from a highly refined carbohydrate diet may thus cause the development of cancerous lesions.

Studies conducted with patients having large bowel cancer support this conclusion. High intake of sugars depleted in fiber and fat predisposes to the development of this condition.[19]

Findings also indicate the existence of a strong relationship between refined sugar intake and Crohn's disease—an inflammatory bowel disease afflicting 100,000 Americans each year.[20] Although studies suggest that it is a secondary rather than causal relationship,[21] the influence of sugar is undeniable. A reduction of carbohydrates and an increase of crude fiber have shown to be effective in reducing the number and severity of attacks of Crohn's disease and extending the state of remission.[22]

Studies also suggest an association between excessive carbohydrate intake and diarrhea, especially among children. In research testing on children with chronic diarrhea, the condition only abated when sugar was removed from their diets.[23]

The increase in the risk factors associated with gallstone and renal stone formation has been linked to dietary substances such as sucrose.[24] A study of Indians and other residents on the Fiji Islands with residents in the province of Natal, South Africa, showed that the Fijians have a higher incidence of gallstone and renal stone formation in addition to diabetes mellitus, myocardial infarction, duodenal ulcer, acute appendicitis and eclampsia (convulsions). Their diets differed mainly in their higher consumption of refined fiber-depleted carbohydrates.[25]

Effects of Sugar in Women and Children. There are additional consequences of refined carbohydrate consumption for women. Breast cancer mortality rates have been linked to carbohydrate-rich diets.[26] In addition, foods and beverages with high sugar content are directly related to the prevalence and severity of premenstrual syndrome.[27]

Studies conducted with pregnant women indicate risks involved with the addition of glucose to intravenous fluids. There were no apparent benefits to the mother, but it was concluded that the infusions may be harmful to the fetus and should therefore be limited before delivery.[28] Incidents of jaundice in full-term newborns were 3.5 times greater when the mothers were given infusions of glucose in water during labor.[29] Breast-fed newborns generally lost more weight, therefore increasing the risk of hyperglycemia, and required longer hospital stays than children of mothers who did not receive glucose-water supplementation.[30]

Children are subject to the damaging effects of sugar even before they are exposed to candies and other sweets. Clinical observations in small children between 12 and 36 months of age demonstrated that continuous use of teething jellies, lozenges or syrups produced hidden fermentable sugar contents in their teeth and gums, although no other form of sugar intake was recorded.[31]

Forms Of Sugar

Sugar comes in many disguises, and we must be alert to its potential dangers in various forms. These include the following:

Corn syrup. Derived from cornstarch, corn syrup is essentially a liquid white sugar with nothing of value contained in it. A large portion of the annual intake of sugar is consumed as corn syrup, which is used to sweeten everything from flavored aspirin to wines and cordials. Presented as a pancake syrup, which "has natural goodness and real down-home flavor," this clear, sticky juice is yet another inferior food. The ingredients commonly listed on food labels are corn syrup, water, algin derivative, salt, sodium citrate, citric acid and artificial flavor and coloring.

Glucose. Also made from cornstarch, glucose is a leading contributor to the adulteration of food. The food industry indiscriminately mixes liberal amounts of this cheap filler in jams and jellies, preserves, processed cheeses, candy, canned milk, store-baked goods and soft drinks. Disreputable producers saturate dried fruits with this sugar to add weight, charging more for the nutritionally valueless extra substance.

Because it is not as sweet as white sugar, glucose is all the more dangerous. People who buy the products listed above may consume huge quantities of glucose without realizing it because they can't taste it. As high in calories as sugar, glucose is in effect a predigested food that undergoes no processing in the stomach or intestines. Back in the 1920s, Dr. Harvey W. Wiley warned that this pure energy source can interfere with natural digestion. The flooding of our stomachs with dextrose (glucose), he said, would create a situation in which the body needed half a dozen artificial pancreases to cope with it. Though Dr. Wiley's battle to ban glucose was eventually lost,[32] consumers saw that they were being misused by greedy manufacturers.

More recent studies have shed more light on the possible dangers of too much glucose. Research involving men and women ages 64 to 87 suggests that the development of glucose intolerance is related to the intake of carbohydrate-rich foods and inversely related to habitual intake of legumes.[33] Additionally, it has been demonstrated in intensive-care patients that hyperglycemia, requiring the administration of insulin, may develop with the intravenous infusions of high concentrations of glucose.[34]

Maple syrup. Can anything that flows from the living core of a tree be bad for you? The answer is yes and no. Yes, maple syrup does contain nutrients, but not enough to make it a healthy food. As with any sugar, there is a tendency to use too much of it, a temptation increased by maple syrup's good flavor.

Even taken in moderation, maple syrup can still be bad for you because most of it is not an uncontaminated natural product. Thirty years ago, the FDA sanctioned the use of a paraformaldehyde pellet to increase the output of maple sap. Plugged into the tap hole, the pellet destroys bacteria normally found there, but which, when eliminated, can no longer slow down the flow of sap during the beginning of the growing season. During this period, the tree's internal chemistry produces growth substances that mix with the sap, giving it a raw taste. To overcome this, a culture of bacteria is added to ferment the drawn syrup and remove the unwanted flavor.

The FDA has established a level of tolerance for the long-lasting and slow-dissolving paraformaldehyde pellets, meaning that a residue of this chemical is now an integral ingredient of most American maple syrup. However, sugarbush farmers in Vermont refuse to use the pellet and the Canadian Food and Drug Directorate has wisely banned its use throughout Canada.

Honey. Throughout most of history, the basic sweetening agent has been honey. Sweeter than sugar, honey is a preferred substitute for white sugar and other sweeteners, because less is needed to provide the desired taste. Hence, fewer calories are consumed. Honey contains about 70 to 80 percent simple sugars; the rest is composed of minerals, vitamins and important trace substances. The darker varieties, especially those left in the comb, contain significantly higher amounts of these life-giving elements.

Pure honey is slightly cloudy with a residue at the bottom of the jar. Most consumers are not aware of this fact, assuming that the cloudiness and residue are impurities. Because of this, many manufacturers heat and filter the honey, destroying some of the vitamins. The clear, brilliant and easy-flowing honey that many consumers prefer has lost much of its delicious flavor and nutritional value through commercial processing.

Bees are highly sensitive to pesticides and they avoid gathering nectar from polluted fields. If they accidentally happen onto one, they usually die before returning to the hive. Therefore, honey is one of the few foodstuffs widely available that has virtually no pesticide residues (sugar cane and sugar beets are both sprayed and artificially fertilized), a fact that should be reassuring but is misleading because other essentially harmful chemical residues are introduced.

Before honey production became a big business, beekeepers used a harmless bee-escape device to separate the insects from the honey saturated combs, then removed the remaining strays with a soft brush. But with the drive for big profits and increased production came the inevitable abuses, and now irritating chemicals are used to do the job more efficiently. Poisonous sprays, including phenol (carbolic acid), benzaldehyde and nitrous oxide, remove the bees, but they may also find their way into the honey. Often, empty combs are fumigated with moth balls (paradichlorobenzene) or methyl bromide, whose residues contaminate the honey as it is produced.

The fact that honey is nutritionally preferred over white sugar does not suggest it is safe to consume in large quantities. It can also contribute to tooth decay, obesity, diabetes and some of the other diseases to which sugar addicts are prone.

Saccharin. The demand for saccharin escalated in the 1970s after cyclamate, another artificial sweetener, was banned. Food manufacturers simply switched to this equally inexpensive sugar substitute and added it to the same foods. Saccharin, a coal-tar derivative 300 times sweeter than sugar, was discovered in 1879. Its chief drawback is an astringent, metallic aftertaste.

Since saccharin is so intensely sweet, however, it is easy to use and cheap to produce. A pill the size of a large pinhead is enough to sweeten a cup of coffee. Anxious to capitalize on these appealing properties, the industry found a way to mask the aftertaste by adding approximately 0.2 percent of glycine, an amino acid.

Researchers reported 20 years ago that saccharin caused cancer in mice, but the product remains on the market.

Aspartame. The artificial sweetener aspartame has become one of the widely consumed sugar substitutes in the United States. Contained mainly in beverages, aspartame is used by many Americans to reduce their intake of the calories contained in sugar.

However, research suggests that to a limited degree adverse neurological or behavioral reactions may be associated with aspartame consumption in chemically sensitive individuals. Elevations in blood plasma levels caused by this additive may inhibit some of the synthesis of neurotransmitters, the critical message-sending cells of the brain. This effect may increase the risk of varying degrees of neurological seizures. Given the results of such studies, the sale of aspartame-containing products should be regulated to warn consumers of possible adverse effects.[35]

Sorbitol. This artificial sweetener appears to be less damaging to the teeth.[36] Tests have shown that sorbitol-containing gum actually reduced demineralizing of dental plaque after foods containing sugar and starch were eaten. One study concluded: "The chewing of sorbitol gum . . . following the ingestion of snacks can be recommended as an adjunct to other caries-preventing oral hygiene measures."[37]

It must be noted, however, that sorbitol has demonstrated some risk to people with hereditary fructose intolerance. Since sorbitol is metabolized via fructose, these risks also pertain to its use. The complications caused by fructose intolerance, which cannot be acquired, have in some instances proven to be serious.[38]

What's more, sorbitol may pose a risk even for people unaffected by fructose intolerance. Studies suggest that sorbitol infusion solutions given to hospital patients may have toxic effects on the liver and kidneys.[39]

CHAPTER 7
Animal Foods

If you still think of meat and dairy products as the centerpiece of a good diet, think again. While animal foods do supply us with protein, it has become increasingly clear over the years that they also subject us to significant health risks. Animal products are high in saturated fat and cholesterol, which increase the risk of heart disease, and they contain an array of hidden "ingredients" that can harm our health. When you consume meat, poultry, eggs or milk, you get food that has been treated with a modern-day arsenal of hormones, antibiotics, pesticides, preservatives and additives.

Indeed, livestock farming has changed significantly in the past few decades. The production of meat and dairy products is big business today, and farmers are willing to compromise food quality for productivity and profitability. Rather than growing animals in natural and spacious conditions, as farmers did in days past, today's breeders pack them into crowded quarters that increase the animals' risk of infection and disease. Thus, the meat industry must increase its use of drugs to combat these infections. Hormones come into play because farmers want to fatten up the animals and get them to market as fast as possible, even if that rate of growth is unnatural.

The results of our modern farming methods, along with a poor food-inspection system, are making headlines for another reason: Outbreaks of food poisoning from meatborne pathogens have been occurring across the country. In addition to containing drug residues, the animal products sold to us in grocery stores and restaurants, it seems, can harbor harmful pathogens that cause a variety of health disorders. In extreme cases, these microbes can even cause death.

The heavy use of antibiotics, for example, hasn't prevented dangerous microbes from invading animal foods. These pathogens include the E. coli bacteria found primarily in beef, the *Salmonella* bug contained in beef, poultry, eggs and other foods, and the *Campylobacter* microbe found in chicken, raw milk and cheese. In fact, the use of antibiotics has led to the development of adaptive bacterial strains that resist specific antibiotics—and these strains can be transferred to the unsuspecting consumer.

Are Animal Products Safe?

To answer that question, let's look first at the rising incidence of food poisoning from pathogens in meat and dairy products. While the exact rate of foodborne disease is not tracked by our government, it seems clear that such episodes are on the rise. As reported in a May 1993 issue of *Newsweek*, *Campylobacter* was virtually unheard of until the late 1970s; now, this germ is the foremost foodborne pathogen. And E. coli 0157:H7, the bacteria that caused several deaths and hundreds of illnesses in the Northwest in early 1993, was not even identified as a human pathogen until 1982.[1]

These types of organisms can cause considerable health damage, particularly in the most vulnerable among us, such as children, the elderly and people whose immune systems are too weak to fight the invader effectively. Contaminated food—both animal and non-animal products—causes the death of thousands of Americans each year. In 1985, the Centers for Disease Control and Prevention estimated that 9,100 people die from food poisoning annually and that 6.5 million get sick, according to *Newsweek*.[2]

Meat products are likely culprits in many types of food poisoning. Animals begin to decay as soon as they are killed, setting the stage for the growth of pathogenic bacteria throughout the process of getting meat to market. At any point in this process—which consists of slaughtering, processing, packaging, transporting and handling in stores and restaurants—meat may be exposed to room temperatures that promote rapid bacteria growth. Even 24 hours of such exposure can increase the live bacteria count by 70 million per gram in sausage, 650 million per gram in beef, and 700 million per gram in smoked ham.[3]

How do these microbes get past our food-inspection agencies? Quite easily, it seems. The inspection system of the U.S. Department of Agriculture (USDA) is highly inadequate because the inspectors simply look at the animals as they pass by, doing nothing to identify invisible organisms such as *E. coli*, *Campylobacter* and *Salmonella*. This system of visual inspection, with its inherent limitations, is all the less effective because it occurs at a fast pace. The *New York Times* reported in 1987 that inspectors examined 60 to 70 slaughtered chickens each minute.[4]

In recent years, the USDA has been running an experimental program—the Streamlined Inspection System (SIS)—that reduces the quality and effectiveness of inspection standards even further, according to *Spectrum, The Wholistic News Magazine*. Under this system, whose goal is to speed up production by 40 percent, only 1 percent of the animals are examined, as opposed to each carcass. Regular checks of products and equipment for contamination have been eliminated, and the inspection time has been reduced.[5]

The difficulty of ensuring meat safety was made all too clear in early 1993, when the USDA selected 90 beef slaughterhouses for surprise inspections and closed 30 of the facilities, citing poor food handling and sanitation. The government's actions were prompted by the illnesses and deaths caused by the *E. coli* bacteria in the Seattle area; all of the closed slaughterhouses produced hamburger meat. To step up the detection of microorganisms in meat products, the agriculture department said it would develop new guidelines.[6]

And it's not just microbes that can get by the government's lax inspection system. Unsafe levels of pesticides and drugs can go undetected as well, and even animals with visible diseases can pass inspection. A 1987 broadcast of "60 Minutes" reported that chickens with visible cancer tumors were passing through the inspection system. According to some food-safety experts, the cancer-causing microbe contained in these chickens is not limited to the tumor site itself, but rather is present throughout an animal's body. Under the new SIS system, more and more diseased animals may make it to the consumer. Says *Spectrum*: "Diseased meat that would have been previously condemned or relegated to pet food, is now approved for consumer use. Cattle with pneumonia, water belly, peritonitis, and contaminated heads are permitted under the new system."[7]

Our inadequate inspection standards are allowing dangerous microbes to find their way to the consumer. But so is poor food handling throughout the distribution chain. Some of these pathogens also deserve a closer look:

E. coli 0157:H7. This bacteria has proved to be especially dangerous in the past decade. While *E. coli* is a relatively rare pathogen, it can be deadly when it makes an appearance. The microbe has surfaced in a variety of meat products, including beef, chicken, turkey, pork and lamb. And in one disturbing case, several dozen people got *E. coli* poisoning from drinking fresh apple cider because the fruit had not been cleaned properly.[8]

E. coli is a tenacious and highly toxic pathogen that lodges in the intestines, where it can cause abdominal cramping and pain, abdominal distension and bloody or nonbloody diarrhea. In a small percentage of people, *E. coli* leads to a serious disorder called hemolytic uremic syndrome, which can cause the kidneys to fail, and even death. Children and the elderly may be especially susceptible to this microbe.

In fact, two tragic *E. coli* outbreaks caused the death of a number of aged people and children. In one of these cases, hamburger meat was the source of contamination; in the other, it was suspected, but not proven, to be the cause. The first incident occurred in late 1984 at a nursing home, where 34 of 101 residents were poisoned with *E. coli* whose source was believed to be hamburgers. Four residents died, while 14 were ill enough to require hospitalization. Researchers found that the organism did not respond to anti-microbial agents administered to the sick patients, and that anti-diarrheal products may have actually aggravated the disease.[9]

The second incident of *E. coli* infection from contaminated hamburgers drew national attention in early 1993, when nearly 500 people were poisoned by undercooked meat sold at the Jack-in-the-Box restaurant chain in Seattle. Hundreds of these people had to be hospitalized, and three children died from the infection. It should be pointed out, however, that only one of these three children had actually eaten the meat. The other two were infected by people who came in contact with the microbe. This tells us that *E. coli* is a highly infectious organism that can easily spread through normal day-to-day contact.[10]

Salmonella. This bacteria can cause severe poisoning and death, and its rate of infection has been increasing in the past few decades. *Newsweek* reports that the number of *Salmonella* poisonings from beef, poultry and dairy foods has doubled since the 1960s. And one particular strain of the microbe—the *Salmonella enteritidis,* found primarily in eggs—caused 375 outbreaks in six years alone, from 1985 to 1991. This strain is especially insidious because it infects eggs while they are developing—before the shell is even formed. Therefore, we cannot avoid it by checking for clean and unbroken shells.[11]

Also troubling is the role of resistant strains of *Salmonella* in the rising number of outbreaks. Of some 40,000 cases of *Salmonella* poisoning each year, an estimated 20 percent, or 8,000 cases, are caused by resistant strains. And animal sources account for nearly 70 percent of these cases. Given the percentage of fatalities attributed to resistant strains—slightly more than 4 percent—it can be estimated that resistant-strain infections kill more than 200 people each year.[12]

It's important to remember that all types of animal products can be a breeding ground for *Salmonella,* and that the microbe can spread via utensils, food processing equipment, cutting boards and the like. *Salmonella* poisoning can come from beef, chicken, cheese, eggs and even milk products. In a 1985 outbreak among infants, the source was a dried-milk product that had been contaminated during processing.[13] And in a 1981 hospital outbreak, the organism was spread from the original source, a package of precooked roast beef, to cold cuts via a meat slicer. Two patients are believed to have picked up the infection from the hospital staff—not from eating infected food.[14]

Campylobacter. This germ has made a meteoric rise in the past 15 years to become the primary foodborne pathogen worldwide. Like other foreign invaders, it can cause abdominal cramps, vomiting, diarrhea, fever and headaches. And, as with other types of tainted animal products, undercooking can increase the risk of infection. In one outbreak of *Campylobacter* enteritis in 1982, 11 people became sick from eating undercooked barbecued chicken at a family gathering in Colorado.[15]

Chicken and raw milk seem to be the leading sources of *Campylobacter,* but shellfish and cheese also can expose us to the organism. Schoolchildren who take field trips to dairies, where they drink raw milk, are easy targets for the microbe, according to *Newsweek.*

Twenty such outbreaks took place in the 1980s during these trips, and hundreds of children in nearly a dozen states became ill from the food poisoning.[16]

Listeria monocytogenes. The number of poisonings from this microbe is on the rise. As reported in *Newsweek*, few people had heard of food-related *Listeria* disease in the early 1980s; today, some 1,800 Americans suffer from it each year.[17] In a study of 154 cases of listeriosis in 1986-87, the Centers for Disease Control found that 28 percent were fatal. Two-thirds of the infections occurred in the elderly or people with a suppressed immunity; one-third occurred in infants. Compared to control subjects, the patients were significantly more likely to have eaten undercooked hot dogs and chicken. In fact, the consumption of these foods accounted for 20 percent of the overall risk of infection.[18]

The *Listeria* microbe grows especially well on sliced chicken and turkey products, according to a 1989 study by the Department of Food Microbiology and Toxicology at the University of Wisconsin-Madison. The researchers tracked the fate of *Listeria monocytogenes* in various processed meat products during up to 12 weeks of refrigerated storage. They concluded that the organism's rate of growth depended on the type of product and its pH level. Near or above 6 pH, listeria grew well; near or below 5 pH, it barely grew at all. Among the foods studied, the worst offenders were processed poultry products and turkey. Next in line were ham, bologna and bratwurst. On cooked roast beef and some, but not all, wiener products, the microbe grew only slightly.[19]

T. spiralis larvae. The larvae of the nematode worm is a veteran microbe that causes trichinosis. It invades the digestive tract, then moves into muscles such as the tongue and calf, weakening them to the point of near-paralysis. The incidence of trichinosis has decreased over the years, as freezers became more widely used and garbage was removed from hog feed. But outbreaks continue to occur, primarily due to the consumption of undercooked pork products. In 1992, for example, Rockingham Memorial Hospital in Harrisonburg, Va., reported that 15 patients had contracted trichinosis from raw or undercooked pork sausage processed by a local producer.[20]

Writing in a medical journal, the researchers state that human trichinosis should be controlled through a surveillance of all commercial swine, as well as strict compliance with existing regulations. The law requires ready-to-eat pork products, for example, to be treated for *T. spiralis* larvae by cooking, freezing or other methods, but the animals don't actually have to be tested for the larvae when they are slaughtered.[21] The end result is that it's up to the consumer to make sure pork products are properly cooked.

Hidden Drugs And Chemicals

The presence of dangerous organisms in meat products is only half the picture. Even more disturbing is the routine use of drugs and chemicals to affect the animals' growth and combat disease. Some 2,000 such drugs—including antibiotics, hormones, pesticides and others—are administered to livestock, and many of these drugs have never been approved for human use. That means we consume potentially dangerous chemicals every time we eat meat products. A government report done in the early 1980s found that, of about 150 drugs and pesticides used in meat and poultry, 42 were linked to cancer, 20 to birth defects and six to adverse effects on fetuses.[22]

People who want to eat meat and dairy products don't have much choice about whether they will take these drugs. After all, meat and dairy producers don't have to label their products with the drugs, artificial flavors, pesticides and other additives used, and they don't have to warn us of the potential effects of consuming carcinogenic or otherwise harmful additives. The drugging of animals is an insidious practice indeed.

In addition, chemical additives in food are implicated in as many as 10,000 cancer deaths a year, according to the Surgeon General's 1988 Report on Nutrition and Health cited in *Spectrum, The Wholistic News Magazine*. Deaths linked to the hundreds of pesticides now in use are excluded from these figures. For each pesticide, the EPA deems one additional cancer death in 100,000 to be acceptable if growers are economically dependent on the product. "The government is sanctioning food growers and processors to add chemicals to the food supply that will kill an unknown number of people each year," states *Spectrum*.[23]

The meats rated as the least safe—based on both the number of chemicals and their concentration—are sirloin steak, bologna, roast beef and ground beef, hot dogs, bacon, pork sausage and liver. Other animal foods packed with chemical residues include whole milk, butter, several varieties of cheese (cheddar, processed and cottage) and ice cream. Somewhat safer are round steak and yogurt with fruit.

Despite the risks associated with animal drugs, the FDA has made little headway in regulating their use. In fact, the agency announced in 1992 that it wants to streamline the drug review process, facilitate the approval of genetically engineered drugs and relax regulations on biotechnology products, according to Michael Hansen of the Consumer Policy Institute, Consumers Union. Writing in the *NYCAP News*, published by the New York Coalition for Alternatives to Pesticides, Albany, Hansen reports that congressional hearings in 1985 and 1990 uncovered serious defects in the FDA's regulation of animal drugs.[24]

The 1985 hearings reached the following conclusions, among others: The use of unapproved animal drugs is not being regulated by the FDA; the methods used to test drug residues in meat, eggs and milk are inadequate; and most approved drugs are not backed up by sufficient data on human safety. What's more, the FDA had not removed several drugs from the market that were potentially unsafe. Hansen concluded: "In a very real sense, antibiotic testing today is where pesticide testing was in the 1960's."

How is the poor regulation of animal drugs a threat to your health? Consider these facts about the various drugs now in use:

Antibiotics. Massive amounts of these drugs, generally penicillin and tetracycline, are administered to animals, both to stimulate their growth and to fight off infections. The problem is amplified because many animals become diseased as a result of the frequently crowded and unsanitary conditions in which they are raised. Rather than preventing disease by providing a healthier environment, many meat and poultry farmers simply use more antibiotics.

The use of antibiotics in animals has grown dramatically since its inception four decades ago. Most animals now receive these drugs. Over four-fifths of all poultry, three-fourths of dairy cows and swine and nearly two-thirds of all cattle are administered antibiotics. In fact, about half of the antibiotics produced in this country are now used in animals, and the price tag for these drugs exceeds $800 million a year in industrialized countries.

The past four decades also have shown us the dangers of using antibiotics in animal and dairy products. Foremost among these is the development of "resistant" strains of bacteria, or those that adapt to the onslaught of drugs and emerge in a new form that cannot be killed off by specific antibiotics. These strains can share their newly tailored immunity with other types of bacterium, and any of these supergerms may then invade the human body through infected animal foods. Drug-resistant strains of *Salmonella*, *E. coli* and the tuberculosis bacteria have been identified in meat and poultry in recent years. All three of these microbes can cause severe illness and even death.[25, 26]

Another problem with antibiotic use in animals is that we consume unprescribed, unlabeled residues of the drugs in meat, dairy and poultry products. These doses, while subtherapeutic, can build up in the body and become a health threat. For example, drug-resistant bacteria may grow unimpeded due to the presence of antibiotic residues. The reason: An antibiotic's job is to kill off bacteria, but it doesn't know how to distinguish harmful bacteria from the "friendly" variety that reside in the body full-time and kill dangerous germs. Thus, the antibiotic residues may eliminate the much-needed friendly bacteria and give the harmful invaders free rein of the intestines.

Consider what happens when a person who is taking a prescribed antibiotic for medical reasons eats meat or chicken contaminated with a new drug-resistant strain of bacteria. The prescription antibiotic will attack the bacteria causing the person's primary infection, but the new strain will go untouched. According to a study conducted 10 years ago, this toxic condition killed 1,500 people in one year alone.[27]

Indeed, antibiotics have become less and less effective in treating humans as their use in animals has become more and more widespread. Other countries—such as Great Britain, Germany, the Netherlands and Japan—recognized these problems in the early 1970s and responded by banning antibiotic use in animals. But when the U.S. FDA attempted to do the same in the late 1970s, animal and drug producers fought to stop the agency—and succeeded. Companies such as American Cyanamid and Eli Lilly, which produce additives for animal feed, have benefitted tremendously from the drugging of livestock and poultry.[28]

To complicate matters, new varieties of antibiotics have come on the scene, in part because some growers want to reduce the health problems linked to the older drugs. The problem with these alternatives—such as the bambermycin used in chicken feed—is that we do not yet know if they will pose the same health hazards. And at least one such alternative, the cheap and potent chloramphenicol, is already known to cause aplastic anemia in low doses. This fatal disease halts the production of red blood cells and can be triggered by only 32 mgs. of the antibiotic.[29]

The moral: Anyone who eats meat and dairy products does so at his or her own risk. What you need to ask yourself is this: Do you want to consume the residue of drugs that have not been prescribed for you by a doctor, based on a reasoned analysis of the type of drug you need, the quantity, the intended purpose and other relevant medical factors? Or put another way, do you want chicken and cattle growers deciding which drugs you will consume? Unfortunately, that question must be considered in your decision to eat commercial animal products.

Hormones. Like antibiotics, hormones are widely used by animal breeders, generally to tranquilize the animals, boost their rate of weight gain and regulate their breeding and fertility cycles. All of these goals are financially driven by a desire to enhance the animals' marketability. Tranquilizers, for example, slow down the rate of metabolism. Thus, the animals gain weight faster and can be slaughtered sooner. Other commonly used hormones, past and present, include the following:

- Estrogen and Ralgro, an estrogen-like compound, to fatten up the animals.
- Androgen to enhance growth.
- Synovex to increase weight gain.
- Lutalyse to synchronize the ovulation cycles of all the cattle in a herd.
- Diethylstilbestrol, commonly called DES, a carcinogenic hormone banned in the late 1970s.

Many of these hormones have harmful effects in humans who consume the residue in animal foods. Lutalyse can affect women's menstrual cycles and cause miscarriages, while androgen is a suspect in liver cancer. In fact, synthetic hormones can cause cancer in animals, which humans then consume. Estrogen, for its part, has been linked to uterine and breast cancer in women and to premature puberty in children. In Puerto Rico, a drug similar to estrogen was implicated in abnormal sexual development in thousands of children under nine years old—as evidenced by early menstruation, ovarian cysts and unnatural breast development in both girls and boys.[30]

The cancer-causing DES is the grandaddy of harmful hormones. The U.S. government banned it in 1979 after four decades of continual use—and assurances that it was safe. While DES is now off the market, its story bears repeating. After all, it's rather disturbing to think that a product could be so dangerous, yet remain on the market for so long. Here's what happened: DES, a synthetic hormone, was developed in the late 1930s and then added to animal feed to promote growth. But the chemical proved to be a carcinogen, and in 1958 it was removed from the feed of poultry—in which its presence was easily detected—when a new law forbade the use of carcinogenic chemicals in foods.

However, the regulations didn't outlaw DES's use in cattle because traces of the chemical could not be detected via existing methods of the time. More than a dozen years passed before it was decreed, in 1971, that cattle breeders would stop using the hormone seven days before the animals went to slaughter. In 1972, DES was banned outright in animal feed, but, again, breeders could continue to use it in the form of ear implants, since the government mistakenly believed this method did not leave residues. Unfortunately, it did. Finally, in 1979, forty years later, DES was banned for good.

During this time, DES also was being prescribed to pregnant women to prevent miscarriages. During the 1960s and 1970s, the teenaged daughters of these women tragically began to develop vaginal cancer. The hormone, it turned out, had a latency period of 15, even 20 or more years. In addition to cancer, it caused other gynecological problems in females, and both urogenital and cardiovascular problems in the male children of women who took DES.[31] In the mid-1980s, new studies linked DES to a greater incidence of cervical cancer and breast cancer in women.[32]

Given the evidence of DES's cancer-causing properties, it's no great leap to question the federal government's slowness to ban the drug and warn women of its dangers. Even in the 1970s, decades into DES's use, an FDA official defended the hormone, claiming that its long-term use in animals had not given "any indication of danger to humans."[33]

Now we find ourselves with another potential problem—the naturally occurring hormones that have replaced DES in cattle breeding. These hormones, including testosterone, progesterone and estradiol, are administered via ear implants to 90 percent of commercial feedlot cattle. But as S.S. Epstein of the School of Public Health, University of Chicago, has pointed out, their residues cannot be detected—as could DES—because the animals produce the same hormones internally. Therefore, the two cannot be distinguished. Epstein believes it is of critical importance to examine the relationship between our long-term exposure to unlabeled, carcinogenic feed additives in the diet and increasing cancer rates. While the naturally occurring hormones continue to be used in the United States, the European Economic Community (EEC) banned them in 1988 to protect consumers.[34]

Pesticides. These chemicals are sprayed on animals and added to their feed to kill off pests. And, once again, their residue can be transferred to the consumer in meat and dairy products. People don't get to make an informed choice about whether or not they will consume an animal food based on its chemical content, of course, because the products are unlabeled. But make no mistake about it, the pesticides are there. A few examples: bologna has 102 pesticide and chemical residues, roasted chicken has 42 pesticide residues, and whole milk has 29 pesticide residues.[35]

Many pesticides are a threat to human health. One chemical, called Vapona, is so toxic that the daily allowable limit has been set at a minuscule .004 milligram for each kilogram of body weight. It belongs to the same family of chemicals as nerve gas.[36] To make matters worse, many pesticide chemicals are stored in the body's fat tissue, which means they can become even more concentrated as they move up the food chain, from plant foods to animals to humans. In a choice between plant and animal foods, a plant food treated with pesticides will offer a less potent chemical dose.

The pesticides commonly found in meat products are cadmium, hexachlorobenzene, carbon tetrachloride and the now-banned DDT (dichloro-diphenyl-trichloro-ethane), an insecticide used for nearly three decades before the government took it off the market in 1971. DDT, it seems, can be stored in fat tissue for decades, causing cancer in animals and perhaps humans as well. A 1993 study from New York's Mount Sinai School of Medicine found that women with a DDT by-product in their blood had a four-times higher risk of breast cancer.[37]

The specter of DDT may continue to haunt us for generations to come. Remember that pesticides pollute the soil, air and water through agricultural runoffs. That fact means plants, fish, animals and humans are exposed to the toxic effects of pesticides and can harbor traces of the chemicals. As just one example, every fish tested in one portion of coastline in the early 1980s had DDT in their bodies.[38] At about the same time, nearly 80 percent of poultry and 60 percent of cattle tested positive for DDT concentrations, according to USDA research. Animals are especially susceptible, in fact, because they must consume about 16 pounds of feed (produced in DDT-contaminated soil) to generate 1 pound of flesh. Again, the DDT they ingest becomes more highly concentrated in them before it is passed on to us.

Additives. Antibiotics, hormones and pesticides are not the only harmful ingredients served up to you in meat and dairy products. Also included are additives such as artificial colorings and flavorings, preservatives, sodium nitrates and nitrites and even flavor enhancers, such as monosodium glutamate, or "MSG." Literally thousands of food additives end up in animal foods.

Many additives can have adverse health effects in animals and humans. Take the synthetic dyes used in all types of food products, such as violet and red dyes in beef and yellow dyes in chicken. Low levels of some of these unnecessary chemicals have been linked to cancer in animals, as well as infertility, still births and birth defects.

More alarming is the widespread use of sodium nitrates and nitrites in a variety of meat products, including hot dogs, bacon, cured and smoked meats and fish, bologna, sausage and ham. These chemicals, once in the body, form nitrosamines, which are potent cancer-causing agents. For 40 years now, it has been known that the highly toxic nitrates and nitrites can cause cancer at nearly any site in the body of an animal, yet the livestock industry continues to use them liberally.

And did you know that two common meat preservatives—BHT (butylated hydroxytoluene) and BHA (butylated hydroxyanisole)— are petroleum derivatives that can cause fatigue, skin blistering, respiratory problems and eye hemorrhaging? BHT and BHA help to preserve fats so that they do not become rancid; therefore, these substances are found in butter, cream, lard, milk, chicken fat, cold cuts, sausage and bacon. Non-animal products containing BHT and BHA include peanut butter, potato chips, shortening, vegetable oils and cereals.

What Price Animal Products?

The meat and dairy industries have been telling us for 50 years, through well-funded "educational" and public relations campaigns, that animal foods are essential to good health.[39] These highly effective campaigns have convinced us that meat and dairy products are superior foods. Not surprisingly, however, the promoters haven't given us the whole story about animal foods' adverse effects on health—effects that have led the American Heart Association and the American Cancer Society, among others, to warn that heavy meat consumption may be hazardous to our health.

A diet high in animal foods has been correlated with heart disease, in particular, and with many types of cancer, including cancer of the colon, prostate, breast, pancreas, kidney and endometrium. Studies continue to verify these diet-disease links. One study, for example, looked at the link between meat and fatal ischemic heart disease by tracking more than 25,000 Seventh-Day Adventists over a 20-year period, from 1960 to 1980. The study clearly showed that meat consumption is associated with the risk of fatal heart disease in both men and women. The link was stronger in men, however, and those in the 45- to 64-year-old age range who ate meat every day had a three-times higher risk than those who did not eat meat.[40]

Two recent studies on the risk of cancer in women also deliver bad news about a high-meat diet. In 1988, researchers reported that daily meat consumption was a significant factor in the risk of ovarian cancer in women over the age of 50, based on a study of 56 such women with epithelial ovarian cancer. This conclusion was true even after the researchers adjusted for reproductive and other risk factors. Nearly 20 percent of the ovarian-cancer risk was attributed to meat consumption.[41]

Then, in 1990, Harvard Medical School researchers reported on the results of a big study on colon cancer in women. The research, conducted between 1980 and 1986, involved nearly 89,000 women from 34 to 59 years old, none of whom had a history of cancer or inflammatory bowel disease. The results: Animal fat was positively associated with colon-cancer risk, and the link between processed meats and liver and increased cancer risk was especially strong. An intake of fish and skinless chicken was correlated with a decreased risk. The ratio of red-meat consumption to fish and chicken intake also was significant. Women in the highest quartile of this ratio had 2.5 times the risk of colon cancer as those in the lowest quartile.[42]

It's worth noting, too, that fatal cirrhosis of the liver was linked to pork consumption by a study that examined the intake of both alcoholic beverages and fat, beef and pork in several countries. The study, released in 1985, found a highly significant relationship between cirrhosis mortality and the consumption of alcohol and pork. In countries where the intake of alcohol was low, the link between cirrhosis and pork was still significant. In 10 provinces of Canada, the pork-fatality link existed even though there was no association between alcohol intake and fatalities from liver cirrhosis.[43]

Despite studies such as these, some people still want to believe that an animal-based diet is better than one high in plant foods, such as legumes, grains, fruits and vegetables. While it's true that meat contains protein, the various types of animal foods may not supply as much protein as generally believed. Fat and water make up 80 percent of the composition of beef, for example, with protein accounting for a mere 20 percent. And the "net protein utilization" rate of meat and poultry, which measures the degree of protein utilization in the body, is 67 percent. The utilization rate is higher for cheese, fish, milk and eggs, ranging from 70 percent for cheese to 95 percent for eggs. These figures tell us that eggs are a highly efficient source of protein, but that other animal foods, particularly meat and poultry, may not be all they are cracked up to be.

Meanwhile, it has become increasingly clear in recent years that "complete" proteins can be formed of plant-based foods. This can be accomplished by combining them in ways that supply the eight essential amino acids in proper proportions, just as do eggs and some, but not all, of the other animal proteins. This development has taken the wind out of the meat-eater's argument that only meat, fish, eggs and other animal sources can supply us with complete proteins.

The scientific research has shown, time and again, that the basic principles of vegetarianism are the very dietary patterns that promote good health and help to ward off disease. These principles have been endorsed in the diet guidelines of major health-related organizations, such as the American Cancer Society. What do they consist of? A high intake of fiber-rich whole grains, fruits, vegetables, legumes, nuts and seeds, and a reduced intake of fat, particularly, of course, animal fats. This diet supplies all the nutrients needed for good health, cleanses the body and helps to provide a preventive shield against the disease process.

In the end, a person's diet is a highly personal choice—and the primary way in which each of us can control the quality of our health and well-being. More than 14 million people now choose to eat a strictly vegetarian diet; many millions more choose a lacto-vegetarian or lacto-ovo-vegetarian approach, which means they eat both plant-based foods and dairy foods. Others will continue to eat meat, despite the potential health hazards associated with such a diet.

In making your choice, keep the facts in mind: Animal foods have been linked with an increased risk of heart disease and certain types of cancer. Vegetarian diets, by contrast, have been linked to a decreased risk of obesity, lung cancer, coronary artery disease, hypertension, diabetes, gallstones and alcoholism.[44, 45] In one 11-year, 2,000-participant study conducted by the Cancer Research Centre in Heidelberg, Germany, researchers found that vegetarians and semi-vegetarians had twice the ability to combat cancer cells. And, compared to meat-eaters, the vegetarians had only half the chance of fatality from circulatory and heart disease.[46]

CHAPTER 8

Tobacco, Alcohol And Caffeine

Most of us equate the word "legal" with "safe." When the government legalizes the sale of certain drugs, for example, we assume that these substances are safe to use. Conversely, when the government prohibits the sale of certain drugs, we assume that they are bad for us. But history has shown us that legal and safe are not necessarily one and the same. A product may be banned from use—as alcohol was just 60 years ago—and then permitted on the market once again.

However, the evidence is in and the so-called "minor" problems associated with tobacco, alcohol and caffeine use have become major in anyone's book. These three legal narcotics account for thousands of deaths every year, and any intelligent investigation of the facts leads us to the conclusion that legal may be more a matter of convenience than protection.

The toxic effects of tobacco, alcohol and caffeine accumulate slowly, lulling many users into a false sense of security because no immediate harm is apparent. Sadly, the deadly potential of the drugs may not be realized until many years later, when the symptoms of cancer, emphysema, heart disease or psychosis appear. By then it is usually too late to reverse the damage.

Advertisers do their best to lure the unwary victim down the primrose path of the addictive products they push. To be well-liked and successful, Madison Avenue tells us, we must drink and smoke the way the handsome, healthy people do in their ads. Advertisements and commercials strive to create the impression that cigarettes, alcohol and caffeine are somehow beneficial to the consumer; the grim reality is hidden behind a smoke screen of seductive, glowing words and images. Let's clear away the deceptions and take a close look at the truth.

Cigarettes And Tobacco

The last 10 years have seen a dramatic shift in our awareness of the dangers of smoking. While we have known for three decades that smoking is a leading cause of cancer death, we have finally acknowledged that secondhand smoke can cause the same health problems as firsthand smoke. In early 1993, in fact, the EPA classified secondhand smoke as a Class A carcinogen. That label means environmental tobacco smoke (ETS) is every bit as potent as arsenic, asbestos and radon in its ability to cause cancer.[1]

In 1988, following years of study, the surgeon general stated that sidestream smoke can be deadly for non-smokers. In addition to causing respiratory problems, ETS is responsible for 3,000 to 5,000 lung cancer deaths a year in non-smokers, as well as 35,000 to 40,000 deaths from heart disease.[2] Secondhand smoke has been determined to be a major health concern.[3]

It is easy to see why tobacco smoke is so deadly. It contains more than 4,000 chemicals, and at least 15 of its ingredients are known or suspected to be cancer-causing agents.[4] But what's truly alarming is that secondhand smoke contains greater concentrations of certain carcinogens than primary smoke. It also contains greater amounts of nicotine and tar, both strong and addictive toxins.[5]

Given these dangers, it's not surprising that many states and municipalities have taken legal action to protect non-smokers from secondhand smoke. More than 40 states and at least 480 communities have passed legislation to restrict smoking in public places.[6] And in the private sector, the majority of companies now have smoking policies that restrict or ban smoking in the workplace. We spend some $22 billion a year on medical care related to smoking (lost productivity costs another $43 billion a year).[7] Even Hillary Clinton followed suit in early 1993, making the White House a smoke-free environment for the first time ever.

But that brings us to smokers. Although the number of smokers has declined in the past 30 years, nearly one in three adult Americans (about 29 percent) continues to smoke. That's more than 50 million Americans, and the death toll among smokers is high. Smoking causes 434,000 deaths a year. The death rate of four other killers combined—alcohol, drugs, AIDS and car accidents—does not equal that of smoking alone.[8]

With all this information, then, why do people continue to smoke? Since 1964, the Surgeon General has warned that smoking is a health hazard. His announcement prompted the U.S. Public Health Service and the American Cancer Society to publicize the dangers of tobacco smoking and offer suggestions to those trying to stop. Cigarette advertising was eventually banned on television and radio, and cigarette packages were required to carry the warning: "May be Hazardous to Health." Later the wording was strengthened to read: "Smoking is Dangerous to Your Health."

But the reason cigarette smokers do not give up this harmful habit easily is simple: Nicotine is a highly addictive substance, like many other drugs. Smokers are hooked as surely as is any heroin addict; giving up cigarettes creates painful withdrawal symptoms and a craving that many people cannot overcome. The Public Health Service has declared cigarettes and tobacco to be our most common form of drug dependence.[9] It is hardly a question of simple willpower. As Dr. M.A. Hamilton Russell, a British expert on drug addiction, has stated: "If it were not for the nicotine in the tobacco smoke, people would be little more inclined to smoke cigarettes than they are to blow bubbles or light sparklers."[10]

This physical dependence has been known for 50 years, since Dr. Lennox Johnston conducted a series of experiments with smokers in his London research laboratories. When volunteers were injected with dosages of nicotine equivalent to the amount found in an average cigarette, they discovered that their desire for cigarettes suddenly vanished. As long as the injections were continued throughout the day, not one of the subjects wanted to smoke. When the injections were withdrawn, the craving returned. Dr. Johnston concluded that "smoking tobacco is essentially a means of administering nicotine, just as smoking opium is a means of administering morphine."[11]

Further proof has been offered by other research, including an important study by the University of Michigan Medical School in the late 1960s. Volunteer smokers were placed inside soundproof isolation booths for 6 hours a day for 15 consecutive days, during which time intravenous needles were inserted into their arms. The subjects were allowed to read and smoke, and they were not told that the experiment had anything to do with tobacco. On certain days, a nicotine solution was fed through the needles, and on others a plain salt solution was substituted. The results were invariable: on nicotine-fed days the volunteers smoked significantly less than usual or not at all.

Researchers discovered that nicotine is carried to the brain via the bloodstream within a minute or two of smoking; it's then eliminated about half an hour later, and the craving returns. Scientists and farmers have long known that nicotine is a deadly poison. They use a concentrated spray of the chemical extracted from tobacco leaves as a potent insecticide. In humans, nicotine constricts the blood vessels, decreasing blood circulation to the skin and vital organs. Long-term smokers tend to look much older than non-smokers—a result of the contraction of the capillaries on the skin's surface, which prevents the absorption of tissue-building nutrients. Furthermore, smokers afflicted with arterial hardening and cholesterol deposits suffer a significantly higher number of heart attacks than non-smokers. Damaged blood vessels give way sooner when shrivelled by nicotine.

Until the early 1900s, tobacco was usually chewed, inhaled as snuff, or smoked in cigars and pipes without being inhaled. In other words, nicotine was absorbed into the bloodstream through the membranes of the mouth, nose and bronchial passages—not through the lungs. The invention of cigarette paper and automatic rolling machinery changed all that, and soon tobacco users were puffing away on convenient, white-wrapped sticks of tobacco that introduced new toxins deep into their bodies. Known collectively as "tar," these toxins are byproducts of the combustion of paper, tobacco and chemicals in tobacco processing.

In healthy individuals, the lungs are elastic rhythmic organs that exchange oxygen in the air for carbon dioxide and other waste gases emitted by cellular metabolism. If separated and laid end to end, the clusters of tiny, bubble-like air sacs (alveoli) that effect this process would fill a space the length and width of a swimming pool.

The inhalation of cigarette tar causes the thin alveoli membranes to break down; thus the lungs lose their natural resilience. Still trying to perform their function of exchanging gases with the blood, these air sacs form larger sacs which tend to trap carbon dioxide. Pressure builds inside the lungs, and it becomes difficult to breathe. In the constant struggle for air, the bronchial tubes and windpipe also lose their elasticity, and the alveoli begin to resemble balloons that have been blown up too long—when deflated they simply wrinkle instead of returning to their original size. This abnormality is known as emphysema, a condition that causes symptoms such as breathlessness, coughing spells and excess mucus in the respiratory tract.

The most lethal byproduct inhaled from burning tobacco is benzo(a)pyrene, a carcinogenic chemical also emitted by automobile exhaust pipes and factory smoke stacks. In numerous tests conducted at universities in the United States and England, benzo(a)pyrene has been applied to the respiratory tracts of laboratory animals, and has usually resulted in malignant tumors. The American Cancer Society identifies this smokeborne substance as a prime cause of lung cancer.

Rather than attacking the small alveoli sacs, lung cancer begins on the walls of main bronchial air passages, whose cells begin to grow erratically after years of constant irritation. If the tumors grow inward, they may cause collapse and infection of the lung, and the patient will cough up blood-stained sputum. These symptoms are considered fortunate, because they are an early warning that the lungs have been damaged. Caught at such an early stage, the disease can sometimes be checked by the surgical removal of the infected parts of the lungs. If the tumors grow outward into the surrounding tissues and no symptoms appear, the disease silently spreads throughout the body, leaving little hope of cure.

The leading killer among all forms of cancers, lung cancer currently claims about 140,000 victims annually. The American Cancer Society estimates that 87 percent of lung cancer deaths could be avoided if only people would stop smoking. And lung cancer isn't the only concern. The chemical irritants absorbed into the blood (including nicotine) are excreted almost unchanged in the urine, and they foster the development of cancer of the kidneys, prostate glands and bladder. Even smokers of pipes and cigars are not immune. Although their incidence of lung cancer is lower, they run the risk of developing cancerous sores in the mucous membranes of the mouth and nose, due to the much stronger tobacco contained in these products. Many pipe tobaccos and cigars are sugar-cured, which further irritates the body.

The most effective solution, of course, would be for the government to ban the sale of cigarettes, and finally recognize cigarettes and tobacco as the dangerous substances they are. Remember, though, that the powerful Tobacco Institute fights any efforts to diminish its commercial interests. It has an estimated budget of $15 to $30 million a year, and it spends that money to lobby against policies and laws designed to restrict smoking.[12]

For those who want to kick the habit, the first step is to recognize that nicotine is a narcotic. Abrupt withdrawal is rarely successful, because the craving can quickly overcome the desire to quit. Many experts advise that the amount of cigarettes smoked should be lessened gradually. One technique is to chew sugarless gum in place of every other cigarette. Then, when the desire for a cigarette becomes overwhelming, draw in a deep breath; most ex-smokers have found this technique to be highly effective. The need for nicotine will abate several days or weeks later, depending upon your tolerance level, and willpower can take over.

Alcohol

Alcohol addiction is second only to nicotine as a prime cause of body pollution. In the United States and many European countries, alcoholism has continued to increase. The number of alcoholics in the United States alone has been estimated at about 8 million.[13] Tens of millions of work hours are lost each year by alcoholics, and 46 percent of fatalities from automobile accidents were related to the use of alcohol in 1992.[14]

Taken occasionally and in moderation, a highball, a bottle of beer or a glass of wine probably will not harm you any more than a piece of candy. Alcohol is an addictive drug, however, and many people find it difficult to limit themselves to one or two drinks a week or month. Before long, many social drinkers find themselves imbibing more and more, and progressing from problem drinker to the ranks of alcoholics, who account for an estimated 10 to 12 percent of all drinkers.[15]

Although moderate drinking is considered to be socially acceptable, even that indulgence carries a social cost. Studies have shown that moderate drinkers have a high incidence of sickness in the workforce and receive fewer promotions. When people stop drinking, it has a positive influence in both work performance and labor-turnover rate.[16] Invariably, social drinkers gamble with their health and peace of mind, since no one can predict with certainty whether they will become addicted to alcohol.

Inexplicably, the FDA views alcohol as a nondrug and permits its open sale in hundreds of thousands of stores, restaurants and bars. At the same time, barbiturates—which produce the same mind-altering effects as alcohol—are legally available only by prescription. In addition, their use has been severely restricted under the Drug Abuse Control Amendment of 1965. Meanwhile, producers of alcoholic beverages spend hundreds of millions of dollars yearly on advertisements that encourage consumers to ingest a chemical that causes even more physiological harm and social disintegration than a drug that has been suppressed.

Like barbiturates, alcohol depresses the central nervous system, producing a feeling of relaxation and moderate euphoria. Similar to a general anesthetic, it numbs the control centers of the brain, releasing normal inhibitions and increasing irrational behavior. One too many drinks has turned many an otherwise sensible man or woman into "the life of the party." Alcohol also decreases alertness and motor ability, as evidenced by the staggering drunk who tries to keep from slurring his or her words. Eventually, the alcohol "high" turns to depression, the brain shuts off, and a dead sleep arrives. In the morning there is the inevitable hangover.

The nauseated, headachy, tired feeling that constitutes a hangover is a signal that the liver is rebelling from a massive assault of alcohol. Excessive thirst is a reminder that alcohol also is a diuretic, which irritates the kidneys and causes them to excrete more water than the body has taken in. Both conditions are evident in the appearance of a hangover sufferer. The puffy gray look occurs because the liver—the major cleansing organ of the body—cannot keep up with the demand to filter toxins from the bloodstream. The dry, mottled appearance of the skin means the tissues have been leached of water and nutrients cannot be absorbed. Ugly red networks of capillaries on the face and body attest to alcohol's strong dilating effect on blood vessels. But alcohol has many more lasting effects. Among them are the following:

Liver damage. Constant drinking slowly poisons the liver cells, which are eventually killed off. Striving to correct the damage, the remaining liver cells generate new ones while the dead cells turn into scar tissue. The regenerated cells form into knob-like clusters separated by thick bands of hard scar tissue, and the result is cirrhosis of the liver. Such a liver is grossly misshapen and enlarged, and often distends the abdomen to form the familiar "beer belly." The risk of developing cirrhosis of the liver increases significantly when alcohol intake exceeds an average of merely 40 grams (1.4 ounces) per day.[17]

Alcohol intake also heightens the risk of non-cirrhotic liver disease (chronic hepatitis). Over a period of 10 to 30 years, the risk of chronic hepatitis is 11.4 times greater among regular alcohol consumers than the general public.[18] Studies show that alcohol not only contributes to liver diseases, but also accelerates liver damage when hepatitis or cirrhosis already exists. Furthermore, habitual drinkers significantly lower their chances of surviving these diseases.[19]

Fortunately for the reformed drinker, the liver is a truly remarkable organ that has the power to rebuild itself even after up to 80 percent of it has been destroyed. But many alcoholics are so addicted they fail to heed the warning signs of jaundice (yellowing of the eyes and skin) and bloody vomiting, and they proceed to destroy what is left of their livers. Death usually comes in the form of a massive hemorrhage.

Often, cirrhosis develops into cancerous cells rather than healthy new growth, in which case there is little hope for recovery. The lining of the alimentary canal is easily irritated by alcohol, and chronic abuse may produce cancer anywhere along the line before the symptoms of cirrhosis are present. The warm sensation experienced when a drink is swallowed is caused by alcohol burning esophageal tissue, and there is nothing beneficial about it.

Another contributing factor to cirrhosis is poor nutrition. Alcoholics obtain much of their daily quota of calories from alcohol, which fuels the body without providing protein, fat, vitamins or minerals. Consequently, they suffer symptoms of malnutrition similar to those endured by people in underdeveloped countries. Among the most serious nutritional diseases associated with alcoholism are neuritis, a painful inflammation of the nerves; beriberi, a vitamin B-1 (thiamine) deficiency marked by an enlarged heart, excessive bowel activity, gastric disturbances and general decline; and pellagra, a vitamin B-3 (niacin) deficiency disease that results in weakness to the point of helplessness, rashes on the hands, arms and face, diarrhea and often emotional breakdown. Because they are malnourished, drinkers have a lowered resistance to infectious diseases, and are inclined to contract lobar pneumonia, which has a higher death rate among drinkers than nondrinkers.

Cancer. Alcohol has been associated with cancer of the liver and colon, in particular, and also with cancer of the breast, head and neck. Alcohol combined with smoking has a synergistic effect, particularly with orophageal and laryngeal cancer.[20] Heavy drinkers show a 15-fold risk of cancer of the oral cavity and an 11-times greater risk of cancer of the pharynx. Combined with cigarettes, the risk is greater than with either substance alone.[21]

Beer drinkers who consume more than 12 beers a month are 1.6 times more likely to contract lung cancer. Although cigarettes are the major culprit in this type of cancer, alcohol, either combined with tobacco or alone, increases the likelihood of developing lung cancer.[22] Among alcoholic drinks, beer also is the most likely to cause cancer of the colon and rectal area.[23]

Women who consume an average of even one ounce per day of alcohol show a two-times greater chance of developing breast cancer.[24] Women who consume larger quantities also increase their risk of developing epithelial ovarian cancer.[25]

Other adverse effects. Heavy alcohol consumption has been linked to elevated blood pressure (particularly systolic),[26] increased hemorrhaging and susceptibility to both hemorrhagic and non-hemorrhagic stroke.[27] Alcohol in pregnancy, even in social or moderate drinking, can induce damage to the heart muscle and cause heart defects in the unborn fetus.[28]

Moreover, alcohol addiction is as destructive to the mind as it is to the body. Years of constant drinking destroys brain cells, resulting in memory loss, hallucinations and paranoid delusions. Delirium tremens ("DTs"), in which the alcoholic thinks he or she sees pink elephants or feels insects crawling under the skin, is another sign of imminent mental deterioration. This pressing problem was investigated 30 years ago, when a presidential commission uncovered the following data: More than 22 percent of all men admitted to state mental hospitals for the first time were diagnosed as alcoholics (the figure for women was 5.6 percent); and approximately 29 percent of male patients in general hospital wards were problem drinkers.[29]

Social effects. Because alcohol releases social inhibitions and lessens alertness and coordination, drinking has become one of the biggest law-enforcement problems in the United States. This burden is also borne by the non-drinking taxpayer, who must daily face death or permanent disability when driving on roads infested with drunken drivers. As far back as 1965, a presidential commission's report showed that about four of ten arrests were for public drunkenness or driving while under the influence of alcohol. Other studies have shown that many murders take place while people are intoxicated.

Alcoholic parents may take out their frustrations on their children by physically abusing them. Research shows that children have twice as great a chance of incurring injuries from a parent who drinks than from a parent who doesn't. If both parents are drinkers the possibility of abuse is higher still.[30]

Like drug addicts, alcoholics are enslaved by a chemical that slowly poisons their minds and bodies while bringing grief and tragedy to those around them. Many people believe alcoholics are skid-row types who have given up family, friends, business and all the other activities that enrich our lives. In fact, they are only part of the problem. For every unshaven wreck of a man, there are dozens of neatly dressed men and women, many of whom drink secretly and are addicted to alcohol. Although they appear to function normally they harm themselves nearly as badly. They are the people who drive while intoxicated, and whose doctors thoughtfully admit them to private hospitals when they become ill to cover up their problem.

A cure can only be effected when a person admits he or she is an alcoholic. Psychotherapy may be undertaken to help an alcoholic deal with the psychological and social problems. The chemical imbalance that alcohol creates in the body—which is the source of the addictive craving—can be eased with nutrient therapy administered by a doctor. Antabuse, a medicine that causes distress when the patient takes a drink, may be helpful as well. The best help by far is available from Alcoholics Anonymous, an organization of people who have conquered their drinking problems and are trying to help others; they provide a list of doctors and psychiatrists who are experts in this field.

Most social drinkers can avoid becoming alcoholics by drinking only on special occasions. If you must drink, stick with beer and wine, drink plenty of water to dilute the alcohol, and eat while you drink. A daily multivitamin capsule is essential, along with a B-complex supplement to replace the amount destroyed by alcohol. Above all, never drink to escape an emotional problem. Seek the advice of a friend or professional help.

Caffeine

Why is that morning cup of coffee so delicious and satisfying? You guessed it—the caffeine in coffee is addictive as well as stimulating, and it satisfies the craving built up by the body during the night. Similar in effect to amphetamines and cocaine, caffeine stimulates the cerebral cortex and speeds up the thinking processes as it defeats drowsiness and fatigue. In other words, it helps you to wake up and keeps you awake.

Contained in coffee, tea, cocoa and cola drinks, caffeine provides false energy for a brief period and increases simple motor skills such as typing and driving. But the chemical action of caffeine is no substitute for the fuel provided by a good breakfast, a fact all too apparent in the mid-morning energy lag experienced by workers who begin the day with only coffee.

Laced with cream and sugar, a cup of coffee is a metabolic insult that places a concentrated burden on the pancreas, which may well result in chronic hypoglycemia (low blood sugar). Immediately absorbed into the bloodstream, the sugar sounds an alarm bell for the pancreas to produce insulin to turn it into energy-producing glucose. Caffeine stimulates this effect, as does the nicotine in a cigarette. An hour or so later, the excess insulin has burned up the sugar in the blood. After an initial burst of morning energy, then, the caffeine-drinker is left with the tired, listless feeling that is symptomatic of hypoglycemia.

Then the morning refreshment wagon brings another coffee and an insulin-producing, heavily sugared sweet roll, and the person is able to make it through to lunch. The afternoon break will undoubtedly add more caffeine and sugar to the worker's disrupted system in the form of an iced cola drink. Eventually, the stimulating effects of caffeine can no longer overcome the debilitating effects of low blood sugar, and the drug merely makes the user dizzy, nervous and uncoordinated.

The same symptoms can appear in a person with a normal blood-sugar level if more than five cups of coffee are consumed daily. A now-classic case of caffeine abuse was reported in the *New England Journal of Medicine* in the 1930s. On the advice of an intern at the hospital where she worked, a nurse began taking a grain and a half of caffeine citrate three times a day to overcome fatigue produced by long hours of strenuous duty. Such tablets were (and are) widely available at most drugstores, and unfortunately require no medical supervision.

Ingesting the equivalent of nine cups of coffee daily, in addition to her four normal cups, the nurse began to suffer one of the most common symptoms of too much coffee: she couldn't sleep at night. Sleeping tablets were needed to put her to sleep and more caffeine tablets to wake her up. The addiction to caffeine slowly increased her tolerance level until she was swallowing five, 10 and 20 capsules in order to function properly.

Finally, trying to pep herself up for a staff party, the nurse swallowed the contents of the box—40 tablets—and the dam burst. "She became confused, disoriented, excited, restless, and violent," the report states. "[She] shouted and screamed and began to throw things about her room. . . . Finally she collapsed and was removed to a general hospital." Unaware of her dependence on caffeine, the hospital staff diagnosed her case as "psychoneurosis, anxiety type, with a hysterical episode," and she was transferred to a psychiatric ward, where she was strapped to a bed to protect her from harming herself. Eventually, the poison was eliminated by her body, and the nurse was able to recount what had happened. Taken off caffeine tablets and coffee, she recovered completely and returned to work a few weeks later.[31]

As you can see, the caffeine habit can become a serious one, albeit not as acute as this classic case. Most heavy caffeine users run the risk of slow-acting permanent damage from years of drinking their favorite steaming hot brews and cold soft drinks. The kidneys are constantly irritated by caffeine's diuretic effect, which can lead to infection and subsequent kidney failure. The stomach lining also is irritated, and gastric ulcers are a common complaint of people who drink too much of this stimulant. Among women, excessive tea consumption is strongly related to the prevalence of pre-menstrual syndrome.[32] In addition, eight to 10 cups of coffee a day make women susceptible to very heavy menstrual flow.[33]

More alarming is caffeine's relationship to heart disease. In fact, studies have found a significant association between coffee consumption and all cardiovascular diseases.[34] In one study, people who drank more than five cups of coffee a day had twice as many coronary heart attacks as non-drinkers.[35] Researchers in

Pennsylvania and Canada also have found proof that a high level of caffeine in the blood increases the amount of cholesterol circulating in the arteries.[36] It has already been established that caffeine stimulation promotes an irregular heartbeat, increases blood pressure and plays a part in inducing diabetes.

Furthermore, caffeine reduces cerebral blood flow, thus increasing anxiety.[37] Animal studies have shown that ingesting high doses of caffeine can have serious consequences, including seizures and psychotic episodes.[38] Caffeine is especially harmful to patients with anxiety disorders. In depressed people, caffeine can induce anxiety, while patients with panic symptoms demonstrate an enhanced magnitude of stress.[39] Even moderate consumers have shown a discernable increase in anxiety with caffeine use.[40]

Pregnant women also need to restrict their intake of coffee, tea, soda and aspirin, many of which contain caffeine.[41] In 1975, the Center for Science in the Public Interest found a correlation between caffeine intake and malformed fetuses in test animals. When fed the amount of caffeine present in 11 cups of coffee, many of the animals gave birth to offspring with deformed heads, missing fingers and toes and cleft palates.

New research also links caffeine with reproductive problems. As with alcohol and tobacco, caffeine consumed during pregnancy increases the risk factor for fetal outcome. Two percent of spontaneous abortions can be attributed to caffeine. This is less than the 11 percent attributed to smoking and the 5 percent for alcohol, but still statistically significant.[42] Women who consume three or more cups of coffee a day during the first trimester of pregnancy are twice as likely to have preterm delivery caused by rupture of the membranes.[43]

Additionally, decreased heartbeat, increased breathing rate[44] and reduction of birth weight in infants occur when the mother consumes high levels of caffeine.[45] Animal studies not only confirm these findings, but also indicate that caffeine may retard fetal development and increase the risk of stillbirth.[46] Newborn infants who were exposed to high maternal levels of caffeine often exhibit increased irritability, jitteriness and vomiting. In many instances, caffeine was found in their urine and the infants were subjected to withdrawal symptoms.[47]

While most parents are wise enough to forbid their children to drink coffee, they nevertheless expose them to the same risks by allowing them to drink sodas, cocoa drinks and tea. The resultant overstimulation often produces symptoms of nervous restlessness that many doctors misdiagnose as hyperkineticism, which is an entirely different condition. Needless medications may be administered to correct a disease that is not present, further polluting the body rather than cleansing it.

Recent studies have linked caffeine to lower bone mass and poor teeth.[48] Drinking more than two cups of coffee or four cups of tea per day may impair the body's calcium balance, thus increasing the risk of bone loss (osteopetrosis) and resultant fractures.[49]

Tea, cocoa and cola drinks contain about half as much caffeine as coffee, but of the three, only weak tea can be recommended. Cocoa contains an additional stimulant, theobromine, which brings the total level of addictive chemicals up to that of coffee. Cola drinks, of course, are loaded with harmful sugar and chemical additives. Decaffeinated coffees are no solution, either, in light of the residues of chemical solvents used to extract the caffeine. Furthermore, all of these beverages contain a number of chemical compounds as yet unidentified, that may also interfere with the body's normal processes.

Recent studies of patients with pancreatic,[50] esophageal and colon cancers suggest that high caffeine intake may have played an influential role in the development of the disease.[51] Tests show that caffeine can increase the glandular output of chemical carcinogens.[52]

Caffeine is an addictive chemical, and withdrawal symptoms often occur with a sudden stoppage of caffeine intake. The withdrawal symptoms include a decreased attention span,[53] slight depression, fatigue and headaches.[54] To compound the problem this addictive chemical encourages many to exacerbate the damage by smoking. The best plan is to gradually wean yourself from caffeine dependence. Reducing caffeine intake means less anxiety, irritability, sleep disturbance and headaches.[55] Switch to delicious, invigorating herb teas (even supermarkets now carry them) or unsweetened fruit juices. After years of being dulled by caffeine pollutants, your taste buds will eventually come back to life and food will begin to taste good once again.

IV

Other Personal Poisons

CHAPTER 9
Pretty Poisons

Once we have polluted our bodies with synthetic foods, chemical residues, harmful additives and environmental toxins, is it any wonder that our physical appearance begins to suffer? A look in the mirror may reveal hair that has become thin and lusterless, a complexion gone dull and ashy and pimples or rashes on the skin. Our bodies are paying the price for our never-ending ingestion of foreign substances, and we are beginning to look old before our time.

The best counterattack to the symptoms of deteriorating health would be a proper diet, exercise and simple cleansing procedures. But most people merely try to mask the damage with cosmetics that contain more dangerous chemicals. In an attempt to restore the appearance of healthy good looks, people rub, pour, sprinkle and spray themselves with cosmetics, unaware they could be making matters worse.

Cosmetics manufacturers—major advertisers on television and in magazines—relentlessly pressure us to conform to fabricated standards of beauty by using products that may be functionally worthless. We may be shocked by primitive peoples who seek to achieve beauty by applying urine to their faces and cow dung to their hair, completely unaware that we are doing even worse to ourselves.

Playing on the fear of social rejection and appealing to vanity, cosmetics advertisers urge people to clog their perspiration ducts with metal salts so as not to "offend" with natural odors; to apply caustic acids to "revitalize" their hair; to paint their faces with multiple coal-tar dyes for the "dewy look of youth"; and to scrub the enamel from their teeth to make them appear whiter.

In 1994, the promise of a shortcut to good looks is a highly effective sales pitch, and American consumers respond by spending in excess of $20 billion yearly[1] to paint, powder and "pretty" themselves. The retail markup of "necessities" such as face creams, foundations liquids and lipsticks is usually 500 to 1,000 percent above the cost of manufacture,[2] which is much less than the amount spent on advertising and packaging the products. Cosmetics companies are in business to promote the illusion of health, and the real cost to consumers is not paid at the counter but in the effects of these products on the body.

The Skin Game

The skin is a multi-layered living cloak measuring about 20 square feet. It contains a complex network of nerves, blood vessels, glands and cells, including the hair and nails. Tough and resilient, this largest organ of the body protects the internal organs, regulates temperature, helps rid the body of wastes in the form of perspiration and thrives on a minimum of care. Toxins in the system show up first in the skin, the appearance of which reveals a great deal about what has gone into the body.

The skin is nourished from the inside out. And despite the claims of cosmetics manufacturers, no creams can be absorbed to any great extent. To maintain the glow of health, you must be vigilant in avoiding the poisons described in this book, and you must maintain a natural, balanced diet that provides all the nutrients your skin needs.

Any unhealthy foreign substance applied to the skin may interfere with its natural processes and cause allergic reactions. Contact dermatitis, the most common, can range from tiny pink spots to red, oozing patches on large areas of the body. Acute reactions, although rare, can occur within seconds of application and result in shortness of breath, heart failure and even death. Some cosmetics ingredients, such as hormones, antibiotics and the highly touted hexachlorophene, have been proven harmful to everyone. You not only run the risk of suffering from an allergic reaction yourself, but of inducing an adverse physical reaction in a friend or mate who may be allergic to what you are wearing.

Cosmetics companies now admit that simple cleanliness and the use of an emollient cream such as almond oil will do more for your appearance than many of their adulterated products. After years of delay, the FDA finally passed a ruling in 1975 requiring manufacturers to list the ingredients in their cosmetics. Here's what you should know when shopping for such products:

Soaps, detergents and cleansing cream. Proper cleansing is essential for a clear, radiant complexion. Dead cells, rancid oil, perspiration wastes and bacteria must be removed daily to prevent blackheads and pimples from forming in clogged pores. By the end of the work day this film of natural detritus will contain dirt, airborne pollutants and, if you wear it, stale makeup.

Soap is the oldest and easiest method of removing surface grime, and it's also the safest. A combination of fats, alkali salts and water, soap has the dual advantage of cleansing the skin thoroughly and then rinsing itself off. Detergents lather better, especially in hard water, but they may irritate dry skin. Therefore, they should be used only by people with oily skin or acne conditions, and even then with considerable caution.

Unfortunately, many manufacturers have chosen to ruin a perfectly good bar of soap by coloring it with potentially harmful dyes and chemical perfumes. To avoid these unnecessary ingredients, choose an unscented bar such as those available in health food stores, or stay with Ivory, which is the closest you can come to an unadulterated product in your supermarket. Dry skin may require a super-fatted bar with additional oils to increase its mildness.

Cold creams and cleansing creams should be avoided entirely. They leave an oily film no matter how well they are cleaned off, which means the skin is only partially cleaned. The basic ingredients of mineral oil, wax, borax and soap or detergents react negatively with sebum (natural oil secretions) and can cause allergic reactions.[3]

Deodorant soaps and hexachlorophene. Until the FDA banned its widespread use in 1972, hexachlorophene was added to some 400 cosmetics, ranging from soaps to vaginal deodorants. Touted as a "miracle" ingredient that "stops b.o. (body odor) before it starts," this chemical destroyed bacteria that converts normally odorless perspiration to its characteristic pungent state. At the same time, the antiseptic remained on the skin, where it slowly worked its way into the bloodstream.

Hexachlorophene was indiscriminately used on every part of the body for years before the FDA belatedly discovered that it caused brain damage in laboratory rats and monkeys and was thus potentially harmful to humans. An immediate concern was the exposure babies had received. They were bathed regularly in the germ-killer by hospital nurses, a practice then perpetuated unwittingly by the babies' mothers.

Manufacturers hastily substituted other inadequately tested chemicals to kill bacteria on the skin. The primary substitute was bithionol, which is closely related to hexachlorophene and has been known to cause skin rashes and swelling. Be very sure to scrutinize the ingredients listed on cleansing products and avoid using any that contain these harmful additives.

Deodorants and antiperspirants. Perspiration is secreted from two types of skin glands—the eccrine and apocrine sweat glands. The eccrine glands, found over most of the body, produce a mild secretion. But it is the secretion of the apocrine glands, which exist in the armpits and genital region, that generates a fetid odor when it interacts with bacteria nestled in hair follicles.

Deodorants are designed to eliminate the scent of apocrine perspiration by killing the bacteria that cause it. The effective ingredients include bithionol and mild antiseptics such as alcohol. Many deodorants also depend upon odor substitution; they use a strong perfume to mask the disagreeable smell. Antiperspirants eliminate odor by stopping the perspiration flow with aluminum salts that swell the pores shut, effectively preventing sweat from reaching the skin's surface. Both of these harmful products are a leading cause of cosmetic injuries in the United States.[4] Danger signals range from itching rashes, blisters and lesions to tiny, hard, long-lasting lumps in the armpits, which are known as granulomas.

To make matters worse, the cosmetics industry puts deodorants and antiperspirants in spray cans that propel the ingredients into the lungs, where they can remain indefinitely. The U.S. Army's Fitzsimons General Hospital in Denver verified this problem when two young women came in complaining of fatigue and chest pains. The doctors discovered that the two roommates both used aerosol deodorants that had badly inflamed their lungs. A rare disease called sarcoidosis resulted and the women were promptly hospitalized. The doctors then found that similar cases had been reported and conducted a laboratory experiment with several popular deodorant brands. Guinea pigs exposed to the various commercial sprays all developed lung lesions.[5]

If soap and water are not enough to keep you comfortable and fresh smelling, then use a natural substance to deodorize your apocrine glands. Try a light dusting of baking soda or a preparation containing fuller's earth, a clay product that can be obtained at your local health food store. Neither is toxic.

Vaginal deodorants. Perhaps the most useless products ever concocted by the cosmetics business are "feminine hygiene sprays," the euphemism for women's genital deodorants. In the 1960s, the beauty trade decided it was time for a genital cosmetic. Before long, women could choose from 30 brands of feminine hygiene products that would "prevent intimate odor."

Most women produce a normal, mild secretion of the external genitals, which may produce an inoffensive odor when the body is confined in pantyhose all day. Normal bacteria act on the secretion and perspiration that have not been able to evaporate. But spraying the delicate mucous membranes of the vagina with chemicals and propellant gases is no solution, and it can, in fact, be dangerous. These substances have been known to cause bladder infection, vulval itching or burning, boils and blood in the urine in addition to other minor irritations.

By the 1970s, the FDA reported that complaints about these products were ten times the rate considered normal for cosmetics. Even so, it refused to reclassify the sprays as the drugs they really are, despite pressure from important citizens groups. If these dangerous products were reclassified, manufacturers would have to do controlled tests to prove their effectiveness and verify their safety.

Given the potential health risks, the best course of action is to stick with the basics. Soap and water are all you need to keep the genital area clean.

Moisturizing creams and lotions. No matter what name they go by—night creams, eye creams, moisturizers, hand creams or body lotions—all such products are intended to perform essentially the same function and contain the same basic ingredients. They are emollients, which means they soften the skin and form a protective layer that holds in moisture. Such creams usually contain mineral oil, lanolin, beeswax and natural oils such as olive, peanut or sesame. These ingredients are fine in and of themselves, but manufacturers then proceed to add dangerous chemicals to these products to prolong the shelf life and add color and attractive scents.

The worst of these is a family of preservatives known as paraben esters. Most creams are not packaged under controlled sanitary conditions, so parabens are mixed in to kill bacteria that may be present. But this fungistatic agent can cause violent reactions, including chronic eczema, crusty lesions, red and painful eyes and swelling of the eyes and face.[6] The perfumes contained in face creams can also cause contact dermatitis. In fact, fragrances of any type should never be applied to the face, which is the most sensitive area of the body.

Oily skin requires no creams or moisturizers whatsoever, but normal and dry skin will benefit from a light application after washing. Lanolin closely resembles natural human sebum (oil), and it has the added advantage of not interfering with the skin's normal activities, such as sweating and eliminating the natural waste products of the skin's constantly replenishing cells. Ask your pharmacist for a tube of ordinary toilet lanolin—which is probably hidden behind a stack of expensive, additive-ridden pseudo-creams—and you will be ahead of the skin game. Or, you can moisturize with Vaseline, which is nearly as good.

"Youth" creams and hormones. Ever aware of our desire to look young forever, cosmetics makers promise us that wrinkles will vanish and chins will no longer sag if only we buy their turtle oil, royal jelly and/or unborn lamb extract. None of these substances has had the least effect on aging skin, however, so manufacturers have suggested a newer, more dangerous panacea—hormones.

Applying hormone-containing cream to the skin can cause severe physiological changes in living tissues. All hormone creams should be carefully avoided until more is learned about the immediate and residual effects they may have on our skin and body systems as the creams are absorbed internally.

Foundation makeup. No makeup is beneficial to the skin, including the hypoallergenic types. A mixture of oils, fatty acids, clay pigments and sensitizing preservatives, foundation makeup clogs the skin pores and attracts pollutants from the air. What's more, you may rub too hard in an effort to remove the makeup, thus damaging the collagen fibers below the skin's surface and hastening the aging process. Makeup also contains foreign material that cannot help the skin in any way and is a potential source of harm.

Medicated makeup is even worse, and its prolonged use can cause significant problems with the body's immune defense system. Used primarily by people with acne to cover up pimples while curing them, medicated foundations do offer temporary relief. However, the ultimate damage they may cause is a high price to pay for a provisional cure. When you apply antibiotic and antibacterial substances to the skin, you build your resistance to them. Then, when the body needs them most, such as to combat a wound or a bacterial invasion, antibiotic injections may not be as effective. Acne can only be helped by a proper diet low in fats and sugars, regular and proper cleansing, and the use of plain rubbing alcohol.

Powder and talcum. Face powder, called "the finishing touch," actually blots out the shine caused by oils in foundation creams. Its principle ingredient is talc, a soft mineral known as hydrous magnesium silicate. Face powders also include clay pigments, zinc oxide and perfumes. Talcum powder is composed of essentially the same ingredients and therefore presents the same dangers.

Talc is similar in composition to asbestos and mined from adjacent veins. It has been found to contain dangerous levels of this mineral.[7] Because it is impossible to use a powdered product without inhaling it, regular users may harbor large quantities of these indestructible minerals in their lungs. An asbestos fiber or talc particle you breathe at age 16 will probably stay in your lungs until you die. Less is known about the long-term effects of pure talc, but asbestos poisoning can result in cancer of the lungs or mucous membranes. It can also lead to slow suffocation from the hard scar tissue formed in the lungs as they fight helplessly to slough it off.

The only safe alternative is cornstarch, an organic substance that can be absorbed by the lungs if inhaled.

Lipstick and rouge. In essence, lipstick is a tube of oil mixed with wax and a coal-tar dye. Unfortunately, it is applied where it can do the most harm to the body. Unprotected by the horny layer of skin that covers the rest of the body, the lips are highly susceptible to allergic reactions caused by the dyes used in most lipsticks.

Cheilitis—contact dermatitis from lipstick—is the most common complaint. The symptoms include dryness, chapped and cracked lips and swollen gums.

The culprits are the coal-tar dyes, which are also ingested into the body. Almost all women who use lipstick must reapply it several times a day because it wears off. These minute amounts of lipstick have been known to cause gastrointestinal upsets like gastritis and colitis. The FDA ignores this fact. While it prohibits coal-tar dyes in eye makeup because they might enter the body, it allows them in lipstick, which has a sure point of entry.

The cosmetics industry tries to justify the use of these dyes by claiming that no one has ever been poisoned by lipstick. But how many doctors examining a patient with blood or liver damage caused by coal-tar products would suspect lipstick? It is a clear and established fact that coal-tar colorings are dangerous to health, and that their effect is cumulative. You would do yourself a favor by either refraining from using lipsticks or purchasing lipsticks made from natural waxes.

Rouge and blush are variations of lipstick. But since they are placed on the cheeks, rather than the mouth, they could be considered less dangerous. Even so, a natural glow is the most beautiful of all. If you feel you must use these products, at least buy those you can determine are colored with vegetable dyes. Large department stores and health food stores stock them.

Mascara and eye makeup. Eye makeup is one of the leading causes of cosmetics injuries[8] in the United States, and mascara, which is comprised of a soap or cosmetic wax with lampblack pigment, is the worst offender. Fortunately, the eye can tolerate little irritation, and mascara users quickly abandon a product that causes smarting, tears and bloodshot eyes. Using mascaras containing "lash extenders," intended to make the eyelashes appear longer and fuller, can have serious consequences. These products contain nylon fiber that adheres to the lashes and can easily fall into the eye and scratch the cornea. People who wear contact lenses are in particular danger of acquiring corneal abrasions and eye infections from these products because the lenses can trap the fibers against the eye.

Eyeliner pencils are sometimes used to outline the upper and lower borders of the eyelids, a practice advised against by the American Medical Association (AMA). The group's files are filled with cases of women who have lacerated the tender mucous membranes around the eye, colored them permanently and impaired their vision. The FDA has reported similar cases resulting from the use of false eyelashes, and at least one instance of permanent blinding from eyelash adhesive has been verified.

Presently, there is no safe alternative to eye makeup. Goaded by the cosmetics industry into thinking they are less attractive without these cosmetics, scores of women continue to put themselves at risk. The next time you're at the cosmetics counter, think again: Isn't your vision more valuable than a temporary exotic effect?

Hair Products

Shampoos, protein and dandruff. Shampoo manufacturers would certainly have the consumer believe that everyone has a problem with his or her hair. Some heads have too much oil, others are too dry, still others are plagued by dandruff and limp hair. One common gimmick is the inclusion of "protein" in shampoos, which the manufacturers claim will thicken thin hair and give it body. This additive is not, in fact, real protein, but rather a protein hydrolysate, which is a solution of several amino acids found in protein. While amino acids have shown some success in repairing split ends of long hair, they are not needed for cleansing and may actually hinder the process. Additional amino acids glued to the hair catch dust at a rate that makes shampooing necessary more often than if the product were not used.

Dandruff, oiliness and flakiness of the scalp are normal conditions resulting from the body's process of eliminating wastes and sloughing off dead skin. Most people who complain about the condition simply don't wash their hair often enough. The scalp will put out an extra amount of sebum and perspiration when the weather is especially hot, we are under emotional stress or there is a lot of dirt in the air. Occasionally, a hormonal imbalance will result in an excessive amount of dandruff, in which case a doctor should be consulted. But for common dandruff, it helps to wash your hair daily with baby shampoo or any type that is pH buffered to match the skin's acid mantle.

Store shelves are filled with an endless variety of cream rinses and conditioners as well. In general, they are of no more value to the health or appearance of the hair than the small amounts of milk or eggs they may contain.

Hair sprays. Once strictly a woman's product, hair sprays are now equally popular with men. The sprays are compounded of a synthetic resin (polyvinylpyrrolidone-PVP) dissolved in water and alcohol. Sprayed onto the head in a fine mist, this toxic mixture is breathed into the lungs and lodges in the respiratory tract, sometimes causing pulmonary problems.

Before doctors understood this condition, they were puzzled by lung abnormalities that showed up in X-rays of patients who complained of breathing difficulties. These people were found to have used hair sprays daily in a small, unventilated bathroom. When they stopped using the products, the condition cleared up dramatically. However the illness, known as thesaurosis, or "storage disease," has increased steadily.[9]

The FDA has received other health complaints about hair spray. These include hair loss, ringing in the ear, headaches and several cases in which hair spontaneously ignited when a cigarette was lit. By substituting a liquid or gel setting lotion for hair spray, you can effectively keep your hair in place.

Hair colorings. The process of changing hair color involves a massive assault on its natural chemical structure. If the hair is lightened, the existing color must first be stripped away from the hair shaft with a caustic solution of hydrogen peroxide and ammonia. Next, a coal-tar dye (also known as an aniline dye) penetrates the hair shaft, swelling it up considerably and making it brittle. Once begun, the process must be repeated on the newly grown hair about every four weeks, which is barely enough time for the scalp to recover from this caustic trauma.

Medical investigators have found that many poisonings are directly related to exposure of the hair follicles to coal-tar dyes, whose cancer-producing effects have long been recognized. In addition, these poisons can seriously damage the liver and kidneys as the body struggles to expel their residues.

Gray hair is anathema in our society, and many men who would not dream of dying their hair use equally harmful substances to attain a "natural" dark color. Called "color restorers," these dyes progressively deposit a dark, flat shade on the hair after several days' application. They also deposit a fine metal dust of pigments that have been found to cause severe irritation of the nasal passages, throat and lungs. In some cases the irritation has been so severe that the tissues of the respiratory tract swelled and blocked breathing.

What are your alternatives to these harmful products? Regular rinses with camomile tea will add highlights to fair hair, and a bath of steeped henna leaves will brighten auburn hair. Graying hair—which is beautiful in its own right—can be brightened and softened by any number of non-irritating blueing rinses available on the market.

Permanent waving. To reshape the hair, the protein molecules must be unbound by a highly irritating chemical called ammonium thioglycolate. This chemical and others used with it often cause serious burns to the scalp and face, and they have resulted in the permanent loss of hair. Occasionally, the setting lotions are splashed into the eyes, where they cause irreparable damage. In one case, where a woman accidentally got permanent wave-set lotion in her ear, the corrosive action pierced her eardrum and caused permanent partial deafness.[10] Swelling of the legs and feet and damage to the mucous membranes also have been reported.

At best, permanent waving will eventually make your hair brittle, dull and lusterless. Instead, use water or a neutral setting agent, such as milk, to set your hair. You will avoid the potentially irreversible effects caused by these caustic and extreme treatments.

Be wary of hair straighteners as well. They tend to break and damage the hair shaft, especially when used regularly, and thus can damage the condition of the hair.

Depilatories. Western women are conditioned to consider excess body hair repulsive, and nearly all American women between the ages of 14 and 44 remove it.[11] The most common method is to shave it off the legs, armpits and arms, but many women also use cream or wax-based chemical depilatories that dissolve the hair so it can be washed off.

The active ingredient in depilatories is calcium thioglycolate, a stronger cousin of the chemical used in permanent waving and even more hazardous. Hair is composed of tissue similar to skin; therefore, depilatories left on too long can eventually cause deep, third-degree burns that may result in scarring. Depilatories should be considered potentially harmful because one accidental spray in the mouth or eye, blending of cream on the lip, or actual tearing of the skin will destroy tissues.

Shaving is a safe solution, although any nicks and scratches may become infected. The safest way to remove body hair is with an electric razor. Apply a "pre-shave" solution first to protect the skin.

Other Cosmetics

Nail polishes and nail hardeners. Nail polishes contain cellulose nitrate, a safe substance obtained from the walls of plants, and butyl acetate, which is a highly toxic synthetic acid. Butyl acetate is a narcotic when inhaled in large amounts, and its fumes have been known to cause conjunctivitis, an inflammation of the eye. Moreover, it can cause nausea, split nails and permanent black stains on the nail beds. The dyes used are not known to be harmful.

Cuticle removers and nail polish removers are not dangerous to the nails or skin, but it's wise to avoid inhaling the fumes. Nail hardeners, however, have formaldehyde as their primary ingredient. This is the same chemical used to preserve dead bodies. Formaldehyde has been known to cause atrophied cuticles, lost nails and damaged nerves at the fingertips. In nail salons now all the rage in New York and other cities, many women are unaware of how toxic the products are that the nail technicians applied.

Brittle, splitting, separated nails often are caused by the physical abuse of hard work and harsh household detergents. Wear gloves when you do housework; keep your hands out of extremely hot water and your nails will improve noticeably.

Dentifrices and mouthwashes. Our nation's high rate of tooth decay is caused primarily by a diet that's rich in starches, sugars and sweet desserts, but low in proteins, vitamins and minerals, especially calcium. All the candies, cookies, soft drinks and peanut butter and jelly sandwiches we consume adhere to the teeth, where they form a perfect medium for bacteria. The bacteria multiply into millions and produce an acid that dissolves the enamel and dentine of which teeth are made.

Toothpaste can help to prevent tooth decay, but the type of cleanser used is less important than proper technique. Toothpaste and even baking soda neutralize mouth acid, but the key is to remove food particles that may build up between teeth. Be sure to brush in a gentle up-and-down motion, paying close attention to the area around the gum line, for at least five minutes. Repeat the procedure after you eat any sugar or starch, and then follow up by flossing thoroughly with an unwaxed dental floss.

Some toothpastes also claim to have a "super-whitening ability."

The only way teeth can be whitened is to clean the debris of food from them. What these products do is polish the enamel so that they reflect more light and seem brighter. Stay away from any dentifrices that make such claims, since studies show that they may contain abrasive substances that wear away the enamel or peroxide bleaches that break it down.

Mouthwashes claim to be oral deodorants, but their only purpose is to mask bad breath with a flavoring oil. Unpleasant breath comes from decaying teeth, food left in the interstices of teeth, or a throat, lung or stomach condition. If this condition persists, it's time to consult a doctor. As for claims that mouthwashes destroy germs that cause odor, the National Academy of Sciences has stated that no convincing evidence exists showing medicated mouthwashes have such an effect.

CHAPTER 10
The Medicine Show

Nowhere is our sad state of health more apparent than in the enormous quantity of medicine we consume. According to popular belief, no one need suffer ill health these days, since anything from a headache to a stomachache can be "cured" with a pill or an injection. Certain drugs, of course, can only by prescribed by licensed medical professionals. These drugs have a high risk of abuse and are closely monitored by the FDA.

However, other types of drugs have been classified as over-the-counter medications due to their relative "safety." They are not as carefully monitored as prescription drugs, and the general public may erroneously conclude that they are harmless. After all, over-the-counter drugs are not prescribed by doctors and are readily accessible in drugstores and supermarkets. Lack of education, advertising and the desire to put off expensive doctor visits may drive the public to seek relief from these less expensive over-the-counter medications.

Nevertheless, let the buyer beware. The hazards created by over-the-counter medications are real and growing. For example: These medications may have insufficient information on the labels; they may omit warnings to patients with certain disorders for which the drug may be contraindicated;[1] or, a consumer may be confused by two products with similar brand names and take one that may be harmful for his or her condition.[2]

The most often bought over-the-counter drugs are analgesics, including aspirin, paracetamol and dipyrone. These medications require special attention due to their popularity. Adverse reactions, although rare, include hepatotoxicity (toxic liver damage), gastrointestinal complications and analgesic nephropathy (kidney problems).[3] In a paper presented by Hadassah University Hospital in Jerusalem, doctors warned that analgesics "require quantitative estimates of the risks involved."[4] In essence, they believe the labeling on these drugs should be improved so people can better determine the level of risk involved in their use.

The elderly are especially susceptible to the improper labeling and dosages of over-the-counter drugs.[5] Unlike the general public, the elderly are more likely to suffer from the symptoms of multiple health problems. Thus, they seek relief from their myriad problems by mixing a variety of over-the-counter medications.

Unfortunately, the elderly are not trained in the hazards of drug interaction. Eager for relief, they may unwittingly harm themselves by mixing different drugs. For example, many over-the-counter drugs contain aspirin and antacids. Aspirin is not always clearly indicated on the label.[6] In combination with other drugs, aspirin may lead to accidental hypothermia and pose a specific risk to asthmatics.[7] Antacids, for their part, may affect the "absorption and excretion of prescription drugs and can alter gastric or urinary pH."[8] These side effects obviously influence drug effectiveness and must be addressed.

Unfortunately, much of what we know about medicine is inspired by the publicity staffs of large drug manufacturers whose prime consideration is to sell their products. Their business is to sell medicine, not to prevent disease and sickness. A wealth of evidence points to emotional stress, faulty nutrition, environmental pollutants and lack of exercise as the chief culprits in heart disease and cancer, for instance. But drug merchants persist in spending millions to search for illusive, if not totally nonexistent, "cures."

The money would be better spent educating the public to avoid stress, to eat natural foods uncontaminated by additives and to get adequate rest and exercise. The body would thus be able to heal itself with its natural recuperative powers, and a minor infection would be prevented from escalating into a debilitating disease. But drug producers turn a deaf ear to the time-proven adage: "An ounce of prevention is worth a pound of cure."

Instead, we are constantly bombarded with advertisements and drug-industry subsidized magazine articles that create alarms so that they can offer assurances. What we are not told is that many of these potions are useless, unnecessary and even deadly. Prescription drugs kill between 30,000 and 60,000 people a year, while thousands more people suffer permanent side effects, such as kidney damage, blindness, deafness and anemia.[9] Statistics on fatalities caused by drugstore remedies are not available, but they are thought to be considerable. Interviews with many pharmacists suggest that when studies are finally compiled there will be a surprisingly high number of prescription medication side effects.

Over-The-Counter Medications

Judging from advertisements, Americans suffer considerably from aches and pains, coughs, runny noses, upset stomachs and constipation. For all of these maladies, we are encouraged to reach for over-the-counter treatments. Pain killers relieve our misery in seconds, sprays open our stuffed-up nasal passages, magical elixirs and capsules relieve our coughs and post-nasal drip, tablets unclog our sluggish bowels and sweeten our sour stomachs. We can buy these drugs without a prescription, much less a doctor's advice.

If left alone and given optimal nutritional input, rest and holistic modalities, the body can do a great deal to heal itself since these ailments are usually more annoying than dangerous. Moreover, by tampering unnecessarily with your body's chemistry, you are exacerbating the illness with poisons that purport to cure it. Your body's self-healing mechanisms will have to overcome the effects of the drug before they can to go work on the malady.

An outgrowth of patent-medicine and snake-oil hustlers, the makers of these overpriced nostrums have been called "the last of the robber barons" by a congressional drug-investigating committee.[10] What follows is a discussion of some of the most widely used over-the-counter drugs:

Aspirin and pain-killers. Aspirin is the most commonly used of all medicines. Tens of millions of pounds are consumed each year by Americans,[11] including its various disguises as a remedy for colds, arthritis and rheumatism.

Generally, aspirin is a safe and effective way to relieve headaches and other minor pains, but it must be used in moderation. That means no more than two tablets should be taken in an eight-hour period. Larger dosages may result in increased blood pressure, rapid heartbeat, vision impairment and other temporary side effects. Aspirin manufacturers fail to issue these warnings; in fact, they are not required to do so. As a result, thousands of users could be poisoned annually, some of whom may suffer permanent circulatory, stomach, intestine or liver damage.

The active ingredient in aspirin is salicylic acid, which acts by raising the pain threshold of the brain. Since pain is one of the body's danger signals, it is always wise to consult a doctor if the discomfort persists. By alleviating the symptom, you may be delaying the treatment of a serious disorder.

Salicylic acid causes stomach irritation in many people, a condition that some manufacturers claim to overcome by "buffering" the tablet with antacids. Such advertising claims are pure Madison Avenue bunk, because all aspirin is alike regardless of what has been added to it. What's more, clinical tests have shown the addition of bicarbonate of soda to be less effective in soothing the stomach than a glass of milk or two crackers taken with tablets. If you must use aspirin, always buy the cheapest "house" brands, because they are less likely to have been adulterated with buffering additives.

In recent years a new analgesic (pain killer) has been marketed under different trade names as an alternative to aspirin. These tablets, which cost as much as 10 times more than aspirin, contain a compound named acetaminophen, which has the advantage of not causing stomach upset. Other than that, the incidence of side effects has been found to be about the same as aspirin, making it a dubious improvement.

Remember that aspirin in large doses is a poison. Children should never be given dosages in excess of the recommendations listed on the bottle. Nor should they take flavored children's aspirin which they may later mistake for candy. National Poison Control Center statistics show that poisonings from children's flavored aspirin are a leading cause of death in the one-to-four age group.

Cold and cough remedies. There is no medical cure for the common cold. No medicine has yet been discovered or created that can destroy the 150 or so viruses that may invade the body and cause a stuffed nose, a cough, muscle aches and a general feeling of malaise. Purveyors of cold remedies choose to obscure this fact in high-powered advertising campaigns that claim to offer "prompt relief from suffering," when their products actually do nothing but add more pollution to the body.

Nevertheless, Americans buy these medications to the tune of $680 million a year,[12] mindless of the harm they are doing to themselves. Most of these drugs are known in the trade as "shotgun" formulas, meaning that they are compounds of three or four ingredients. The first is usually aspirin, the second a decongestant, the third an antihistamine, and the fourth may be ascorbic acid (vitamin C) or an antacid.

Decongestants reduce swelling of the membranes in the nose and upper respiratory tract and temporarily alleviate the stuffed-up feeling of a cold. But the membranes soon swell up again and the clogged feeling returns, so sufferers take another dose. The result is a condition called "rebound congestion," a swelling worse than the original one. Nasal sprays should be avoided, because they all contain decongestants and are breeding grounds for bacteria. The spray tip is contaminated every time the user puts it into his or her nose. Within a few days, millions of bacteria have multiplied in the fluid and are ready to repeat the infection.

Antihistamines are of equally dubious value. When an allergic reaction occurs, the body secretes histamines, defensive substances that can result in a runny nose and watery eyes. Antihistamines block this natural action only too well, and often the mucous membranes of the respiratory system dry out and a cough is brought on. At the very least antihistamines will make you drowsy, which is why they are also used as the active ingredient of over-the-counter sleeping tablets.

Coughing is a reflex response to an irritation anywhere in the lungs or the respiratory tract, and often accompanies a cold. More than 800 nonprescription cough medicines are available to the unwary, and most contain the same ingredients. Cough suppressants and expectorants are added to the mixture, further defeating the natural function of a cough, which is to bring up thick mucous secretions clogging the lungs and throat.

The only health-promoting ingredient in any of these preparations is vitamin C, which is included in such tiny amounts as to be virtually useless. The FDA has concluded that most of these remedies, in their present combinations, are not only ineffective, but also a danger to health. A healthy, clean body will forestall most viral attacks, but if you do succumb to a cold, the best treatment is get plenty of rest, drink a lot of water, drink five vegetable juices a day and consume adequate amounts of vitamin C and garlic. It is also important to eliminate stress, which causes the body's autoimmune system to break down, making you more susceptible to viruses and infections. A hard candy or a honey drop will do more to soothe your throat than the most expensive lozenge.

Laxatives. Despite the prompting of television commercials, "irregularity" is no reason to take a laxative. Individual bowel habits vary substantially, and no one can accurately define what constipation is. In a healthy person, nature always takes care of the elimination of waste matter from the body. This usually occurs at daily intervals, but it is not imperative that it does. Conditions such as dehydration may cause the skipping of bowel movements for a day. It is nothing to worry about; nature will eventually cause the intestines to evacuate the accumulated waste material.

Some people regularly consume laxatives in the mistaken belief that waste matter in the intestine is poisonous and must be eliminated from the body as soon as possible. Waste matter is made up of undigested food, broken down blood cells and other body debris. The toxins that occur in the body are taken into the intestine for elimination, but this is a one-way process and normally the toxins do not reenter the body.

True, constipation can occur in people who are bedridden or afflicted with severe emotional problems, in which case a doctor should be consulted. Hard stools and difficult passage are not symptoms of true constipation, but rather of a diet lacking in roughage. Add more fiber-rich foods to your meals, including bran, wheat germ, raw vegetables and unpeeled fruit, and you will find that bowel movements are both easier and more frequent. Laxatives only make matters worse by depleting the body of potassium, hence causing muscle weakness and requiring another harsh dose of laxative to get the bowels to work.

Antacids. Antacids are nearly as popular as aspirin. They are advertised as an antidote to the catchall malady called "indigestion." The word has no medical meaning, but is used to refer to many different irritations of the stomach. Nausea, gas, a bad cold, escape of acid into the esophagus ("heartburn") and emotional distress can all produce similar symptoms.

Treating oneself with antacids is a risky proposition, since an upset stomach may be an indication of a more serious illness, such as ulcers or even cancer. Any chronic case of indigestion should be brought to a doctor's attention, not self-diagnosed. Many people who thought they had eaten something that didn't agree with them never lived to find out that their gastric upset was actually the first symptom of a coronary heart attack.

For these reasons, antacids should be avoided and the cause of the indigestion determined by a doctor. In any event, they should never be taken for a long period of time, because the active ingredient of calcium carbonate may form stones in the kidneys and cause irreparable damage. A glass of warm milk is the safest antidote to occasional stomach distress.

For people who have mild kidney impairment, antacids may pose a special problem. According to one study, four such patients who took daily over-the-counter antacids containing four to eight grams of calcium became severely hypercalcemic (excess calcium in the blood). The researchers concluded that these medications should include dosage warnings to avoid this serious problem.[13]

Boric acid. Once a common item in medicine cabinets, boric acid powder is one of the most lethal poisons ever available in drugstores. While it has mild germ-killing properties when dissolved in water and used as a lotion, boric acid powder can cause severe reactions if applied directly to cut or abraded skin. Inhaled, the powder is an acute irritant of the central nervous system, and in sufficient quantities it can cause death.

The AMA has repeatedly urged the FDA to ban this poisonous drug, but the agency does not consider boric acid to be a poison because it is labeled "for external use only." However, there have been numerous cases of infant death caused by an external dusting with boric acid powder. In one such case, a father put nine ounces of boric acid on the diapers of his nine-month-old daughter. She died one day later of severe damage to the intestinal tract.

Prescription Medicine

Many of the drugs introduced in the past 50 years promised a revolution in medicine. With the discovery of antibiotic "wonder" drugs, the public could be cured of ailments that had formerly been disabling or even fatal. Various hormones offered relief from glandular, skin, bone and blood disorders, as well as the most effective means of birth control yet devised. Chemicals enabled us to control anxiety, they put us to sleep, and gave us energy when we awoke.

According to the drug industry, the millennium was at last at hand and only death remained to be conquered. Then doctors began to notice a frightening phenomenon: The cure was often worse than the disease. Many of these miracle cures had so many dangerous and even fatal side effects that they spawned a new malady called iatrogenic disease, meaning a health ailment caused by medicines.

In their haste to earn enormous profits, some irresponsible drug manufacturers foisted (and continue to do so) inadequately tested drugs on a gullible public, and tens of thousands of innocent people die or are impaired annually. Because many doctors rely heavily on drug therapy and prescribe too many drugs too often, it is imperative that the layman be alert to the dangers of the following medications.

Antibiotics. For all their undisputed benefit to mankind, antibiotics remain a double-edged sword. Penicillin and its 100 or so cousins are remarkably effective cures for a variety of diseases caused by microbes including pneumonia, scarlet fever, typhoid, tetanus and venereal disease. Injected under the skin or taken orally, antibiotics swiftly attack and kill germs, funguses and some viruses, while leaving human tissue alone.

On the down side, however, antibiotics also destroy many strains of bacteria normally present in the body. Ordinarily, these strains compete with each other and their numbers are kept in check. When an antibiotic is administered, most of these bacteria perish along with the infection, leaving one or two strains to proliferate without competition. The bacteria explode in numbers, toxins overwhelm the body and the result is one of the most feared hazards of antibiotic therapy—superinfection, which is fatal in 30 to 50 percent of cases.[14]

Many people also are allergic to antibiotics, especially penicillin. Upon injection, the patient may go into anaphylactic shock, fall into a coma and die. Adrenaline must be given within minutes as an antidote. Some antibiotics produce permanently debilitating side effects, a startling fact soft-pedaled by the drug industry. Streptomycin may cause deafness and permanent loss of balance, and chloramphenicol may injure bone marrow, causing chronic anemia.

The cover story in an April 1993 *Newsweek* declares the end of antibiotics' effectiveness, at least as a so-called miracle drug. In part because of indiscriminate overprescribing, antibiotics have lost much of their ability to combat bacteria. Heavily dosed over the years, bacteria have begun to build up a resistance to antibiotics, and new strains are evolving that do not respond to antibiotic therapy. Twenty years ago, a congressional committee placed the blame for this problem squarely on the shoulders of drug producers who push antibiotics to physicians, who in turn overprescribe them. Most of us already have enough antibiotics coursing through our systems from eating livestock fed with them to promote growth. Constant exposure to antibiotics has given lethal microbes the means to mutate into new forms, while sensitizing us into allergic reactions.

Never use an antibiotic unless absolutely necessary to save your life, or to cure an otherwise hopeless condition. Always demand an allergy test, and ask your doctor about the specific possible side effects.

Steroid hormones. None of this group of widely publicized drugs cures disease. They act by reducing painful and aggravating symptoms in ways not yet clearly understood. Cortisone is the most-used steroid hormone and, like the others, it is a chemical that reproduces a secretion of the adrenal glands. Cortisone and its companion steroid, ACTH, can be remarkably effective in relieving symptoms of arthritis, rheumatism, skin and blood disorders and even some types of cancer.

Undesirable and serious side effects often interfere with treatment, however, and steroids are not the panacea doctors once believed them to be. The most common problem related to hormone use is water retention, leading to tissue swelling (edema) and high blood pressure. As additional hormones interfere with the body's natural metabolism, any number of seemingly unrelated conditions can result, including ulcers, osteoporosis (thinning of the bones), diabetes and psychosis that mimics insanity.

With long-term treatment, the adrenal glands shrink and the body is unable to produce its own hormones once the drug is stopped. In case of accident or an operation, the patient's own adrenal glands may not be able to withstand the stress.

Tranquilizers. Thanks to a massive advertising campaign, tranquilizers are among the most prescribed drugs in the United States. Nearly as familiar as aspirin, tranquilizers are promoted as happiness pills that do everything from "restoring the zest for living" to "controlling anxiety, tension, irritability and depression." In other words, you don't need to deal with the stresses of life in constructive and appropriate ways. All you have to do is pop a pill to erase them.

Such claims may well be mere advertising puffery, judging from tests conducted by the Veteran's Administration and the National Institute of Mental Health. In this study, half the participants took the active drug, while the others took placebos (dummy tablets). The tests were "double-blind," meaning that neither the doctors who administered the pills nor patients knew which was which.

The subjects were examined before and after the experiment so that the results could be judged objectively and not on the basis of what the volunteers thought they felt. After six weeks, half the patients given tranquilizers showed a marked decline in nervousness, tension, irritability and so on. But so did nearly half the patients who took placebos. The researchers concluded: "[Tranquilizers] generally come out as being a little better than a placebo, but not by any dramatic margin."

No evidence exists to support the extravagant claims made by the manufacturers of these useless drugs, which seem to work because patients expect them to. Yet their price is steep: At one point, the wholesale price of one leading tranquilizer was 30 times the official price of gold.[15] A glass of warm milk or a cup of camomile tea will relax you as effectively.

Sleeping pills. From time to time most of us experience difficulty in falling asleep or staying asleep. Usually, the cause is an especially tense day at home or at the office, or drinking coffee, tea or cola drinks close to bedtime. Missing a few hours of sleep will not have an adverse effect on health, and the next night you will probably sleep quite well.

But pharmaceutical companies are not content to let well enough alone. They urge us to take sleeping tablets for a "deep, natural sleep." This claim is totally misleading, since barbiturates and their synthetic substitutes simply knock us out. A barbiturate-induced sleep results from a massive depressant assault on the central nervous system and the spinal cord. Tolerance to the drug quickly builds and before long, a larger dosage is needed to lull us into an unconsciousness that passes for sound sleep. Because the drug is a narcotic, addiction could occur.

Those addicted to sleeping tablets closely resemble alcoholics, in that they slur their words, appear to be confused and generally look unhealthy due to the poisoning of their tissues. Drinking alcohol with barbiturates and other sleeping potions can easily result in death from suffocation, and is a not uncommon occurrence. Unable to resume a natural sleeping pattern, the chronic user may become impatient when the usual dose fails to work. He or she then swallows several more tablets. In this intoxicated state, the person may forget how many doses he or she has taken, and the tragic result often is unintentional suicide.

Those who try to kick the habit may suffer needlessly. The withdrawal symptoms are more severe than those of a heroin addict, and they include paranoid delusions, hallucinations, fever, violent tremors and epileptic seizures.

The toxic effects of key ingredients such as ethylendiamines include nausea, vomiting, blurred vision, tremors and constipation.[16] Sleep aids also contain ingredients such as bromides, methapyrilene, scopolamine and pyrilamine. These ingredients affect the central nervous system and can cause serious side effects in the unwary consumer, including delirium, coma and at times death in children and adults.[17] To make matters worse, manufacturers frequently change proportions and mixtures in these products.

Amphetamines. Commonly known as "speed," amphetamines began to be widely abused in the 1960s. They were originally designed to treat a rare but serious disease, narcolepsy (uncontrollable sleep), but their use soon spread due to the drug industry's high-pressure sales techniques. Manufacturers promoted the drug as an appetite-suppressant to counter the growing national problem of obesity. Before long, teenaged students were snatching Mom's diet pills because they seemed to keep them alert during all-night "cram" sessions before tests.

Indeed, the drug did stimulate alertness, as well as induce a euphoric high when injected. Demand grew throughout the 1960s and drug manufacturers increased production, seemingly oblivious to the fact that a large proportion of amphetamines were being diverted into the black market for thrill-seekers. Gradually, the corroded underside of the golden pill came to light. Emaciated, unkempt and sickly, "speed freaks" were a familiar sight in youth ghettos across the country, attesting to the mind and body destroying power of amphetamines.

Although not physically addictive, amphetamines encourage psychological dependency. Using them to obtain more energy only depletes the body of essential nutrients, and you will pay later in the form of illness or a psychotic mental state. Unlike foods, amphetamines offer no energy; they draw from existing reserves. Withdrawal usually results in severe depression that drives many back to the drug or to suicide, complete exhaustion, paranoia, aggressiveness and brain damage. Deaths from heart failure have occurred among athletes who mistakenly tried to increase their endurance by using amphetamines.

The FDA finally imposed severe restrictions on the manufacture and distribution of amphetamines in 1972, effectively drying up the black market. The drugs are, however, still available on prescription and many doctors are willing to prescribe them indiscriminately.

The pill and estrogen hormones. Oral contraceptives prevent pregnancy by inhibiting the release of new eggs (ovulation). The pill is a combination of two female hormones, progesterone and estrogen. It induces a state similar to pregnancy, when it is impossible to be re-impregnated. For this reason, morning sickness, nausea and swelling of the breasts often accompany the contraceptive effect.

More important, the pill can also cause blood clots in the legs, high blood pressure, vaginal infections, fluid retention and weight gain. Doctors long suspected that the pill caused circulatory problems that could prove fatal, but it wasn't until 1975 that statistics offered irrefutable proof. Then, a study by Planned Parenthood revealed that oral contraceptives are relatively safe for women up to the age of 30, but that risk of adverse effects increases substantially with age. Between the ages of 30 and 40, complications occur often, and over age 40, use of the pill presents a definite hazard to health.[18]

Women in the 40-plus age group may suffer from blood clots, strokes and heart attacks directly related to oral contraceptives. Factors such as obesity, smoking, diabetes and high blood pressure can complicate the risk. Women in this age group are advised to use safe contraceptive methods, such as condoms and diaphragms.

Drugs and pregnancy. The mother-to-be should avoid all unnecessary medications, lest damage result to the fetus. Aspirin increases the risk of brain damage, barbiturates have been known to cause bleeding in newborn babies, and antihistamines may produce breathing difficulties.

Perhaps the most tragic example of drugs that harm fetuses is diethylstilbestrol (DES), which was widely administered to pregnant women in the 1960s to prevent miscarriage. The hormone worked remarkably well and many children were born as a result, with no harmful side effects to the mothers. Strangely, when the female children reached adolescence, many of them developed a rare but deadly form of cervical cancer. Drug manufacturers had not conducted adequate laboratory tests, and in their haste had not even considered possible toxic effects on the unborn.

It wasn't until 1962 that medical science finally dispelled the myth that the placenta—the protective sac that surrounds the fetus in the uterus—prevented dangerous substances from reaching the child. That year, newspaper headlines worldwide revealed just how much that knowledge had cost. Drug companies had promoted and sold a drug to relieve the discomforts of pregnancy, which actually caused a malformation of fetal arms and legs, making them resemble the flippers of seals. The name of the drug was thalidomide, which was developed by a West German pharmaceutical company, Chemie Grunenthal, in the 1950s.

A U.S. company obtained the rights to manufacture and market the drug here, but thalidomide never made it to the American market due to the efforts of Dr. Frances Kelsey of the FDA, who did not believe the studies on the drug proved it was safe for human consumption. When *Time* reported in 1962 that thousands of infants had been born in West Germany and England without arms or legs, or with flipper-like appendages, Dr. Kelsey emerged as a hero. Her courage and intelligence had saved many Americans from a tragic nightmare.

Human Guinea Pigs

Sadly, the drug industry and the FDA are not always effective watchdogs. When a new drug is put on the market, the consumer often is the guinea pig who must test its safety. One drug launched in 1960, known as MER/29, was meant to lower blood cholesterol. But within months it was apparent that MER/29 did more harm than good. Some patients developed ichthyosis (fishlike skin), a painful itchy malady, while others lost their hair or developed a permanent cataract blindness. Information submitted by the drug maker, the William S. Merrell Co., was discovered to have been falsified, and three executives were fined and sentenced to six months' probation. In civil suits, Merrell paid as much as $55 million to those harmed by MER/29.

The list goes on. Chymopapain, an injected drug that purported to repair slipped discs without surgery, was finally rejected by the FDA after it had been used on more than 14,000 patients, several of whom died as a result. Serc, invented by Unimed, Inc., was claimed to be the first effective cure of Meniere's Syndrome, a progressively worsening condition of the inner ear that causes dizziness and hearing loss. The FDA seemed about to approve it when the Consumer's Union brought suit.[19] Serc was found to aggravate the symptoms of Meniere's Syndrome, and plans for its manufacture were dropped.

How do these drugs get through to the public? In part, it is because physicians are overwhelmingly busy and cannot keep up with the flood of medical literature. Therefore, they may not be aware of the dangers of a drug they are prescribing. Also, too many doctors believe drug makers' literature and place a lot of faith in the company's scientists, believing that the ethics of science preclude dishonesty on the part of a pharmaceutical researcher.

Ultimately, it is the responsibility of the FDA to protect us from dangerous drugs. But some harmful medications do indeed make it onto the market, and individual consumers would do well to become as knowledgeable as possible about the potential effects of any drug they take, whether it is prescribed by a doctor or purchased over the counter in a drug store. In the latest medical disaster, tens of thousand of women who had silicone breast implants are worrying whether or not they have biological time bombs ticking away in their bodies. The three million dollar settlement is not of much consolation to those whose immune systems are permanently, adversely effected.

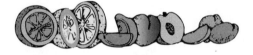

PART TWO

CLEANSING AND REBUILDING YOUR BODY

Detoxification

CHAPTER 11

Getting The Poisons Out
Of Your Body

The toxins in our environment are so pervasive that the task of defending the body against them may seem overwhelming. As always, though, the individual can gain the most control over his or her health through the simple measures that we take for granted. The most important of these is our diet. With every meal you eat, you make a choice about whether you will nourish the body with essential nutrients or deny it the fuel it needs to promote good health and ward off the disease process.

There is certainly a great deal of interest these days in how we can go about making salutary dietary changes. And for those of us who are interested in making such changes—eliminating meat from our diets, reducing dairy products and total fats and sugars, and increasing our intake of fresh, organically grown vegetables and fruits—numerous outstanding cookbooks are available for guidance and inspiration.

As we make a healthy dietary transition, some of us may become interested in looking beyond diet, to the topic of natural healing.

Therefore, in the pages that follow we look at a variety of natural healing practices, as explained by their practitioners. Hundreds of books have been written on natural healing and folk remedies, and traditionally, when one considers the whole of our country's history, the average American has used natural remedies. Today, the scope of natural healing is broad. Some of the practices included within it are: herbal remedies; raw food diets; macrobiotic diets; fasting; water therapies; esoteric energy therapies, such as reiki and rolfing; kinesiology; massage; meditation; yoga; aroma therapy; and homeopathy.

It is not the purpose of this book to examine every alternative healing system, but rather to support a view that the body has substantial healing, regeneration, and self-cleansing powers if given proper physical, mental and spiritual support to use these. Because the average person is not as likely to seek out an esoteric healing system such as reiki we've placed emphasis on guidance from the doctors who practice this medicine.

With this in mind, and in a spirit of intellectual exploration, let us meet two of the practitioners of the esoteric approaches to health that are being offered today.

William Philpott, M.D.
A Comprehensive Approach

Dr. Philpott explains that vitamin C, as a reducing agent, ties up toxins. As you withdraw from a food or chemical, he says, you can handle the accompanying symptoms by eating enough vitamin C. "In my practice, when people are going through food withdrawal, I always administer intravenous vitamin C, anywhere from 25 to 50 grams."

At home, you can take bowel-tolerated doses orally. Every three to four hours take a teaspoon of vitamin C, up to the point of diarrhea. Then, back off to a dose just slightly below that amount. Dr. Philpott explains that this will help you handle many of the symptoms you will experience as you withdraw from allergy-producing, addictive, or otherwise toxic substances. All of these reactions—allergic, addictive, and nonimmunologic—are acidifying to the body. The acid interferes with the body's processing through the cells of its energy system, and we need a buffer against the acid. Vitamin C, in the form of sodium ascorbate, will help this; it's really alkalizing as well as reducing in nature.

Food And Chemical Reactions

Vitamin C is just part of Dr. Philpott's multifaceted approach to detoxification. In his book *Health Strategies*, he goes into detail about how people can help detoxify themselves and overcome food and chemical reactions. He explains that food reactions stem from three basic causes: one is true allergy with antibodies; another is a non-immunologic maladaptive reaction related to a deficiency, such as an enzyme or a hormonal deficiency. In essence, nutritional deficiencies are precursors to these things. The third cause is addictive withdrawal.

Dr. Philpott advocates a method of detoxification and of identifying and overcoming food and chemical reactions that involves five days of eating infrequent foods. He does caution that there are certain groups of people who should not try this method: those who have seizures—because it might precipitate seizures—and diabetics on insulin. Except for diabetics and hypoglycemics, he says that a good food to eat during these five days is watermelon, which is loaded with minerals and water. "Go on a watermelon fast if you like. You may eat fish as well during this period to keep your protein content up, although salmon and tuna should not be eaten. Beef and chicken should definitely be avoided. Too many people react to those foods during the withdrawal phase." Extra vitamin C may be helpful during this phase.

After this period, you simply proceed with test meals of single foods, says Dr. Philpott. If you get a symptom, you'll know it within an hour. At night you can take a couple of teaspoons of vitamin C as an ascorbate, although you wouldn't do that during the day because it would interfere with your testing. In a period of 30 days you can clear up your food reactions.

"At the same time, " says Dr. Philpott, "avoid common chemical contacts—such as car exhaust, perfumes and lipsticks—by isolating yourself from your usual chemical environment. It takes longer—about 21 days—to get these things out of your fat cells. Tobacco, for example, contains fat-soluble materials. You are not going to be over your withdrawal phase from tobacco in five days. But with water-soluble items that are in most of your foods—you can reverse the situation in that time. If you follow this program you'll be in pretty good shape by the end of one month.

"Then you can start your four-day diversified rotation diet, leaving out the food you are reacting to initially and putting it back into your diet in about three months. Most of the time there won't be any problem, as long as you rotate the food in your diet."

Heavy-Metal Detoxification

A person with heavy-metal toxicity should undergo EDTA chelation, which is a recognized treatment for heavy-metal toxicity and can even be paid for through insurance. The person giving you chelation therapy is also likely to give you intravenous vitamin C.

Dr. Philpott says that at home, those bowel-tolerated doses of vitamin C would gradually process the toxins out of your body anyway. But if you're not going to take bowel-tolerated doses, you can take up to a teaspoon of sodium ascorbate at night.

Don't be concerned about a loose stool resulting from vitamin C, says Dr. Philpott. "That's not harmful at all. In fact, I think everyone would do well to take at least a teaspoon three times a day—that's 12 grams of vitamin C orally—every day of their life. I've tested the bowel-tolerated doses of a lot of people. In some of our patients we had to get up to 30 grams a day before they spilled any into their urine at all. In other words, they used it all to tie up their toxins. Twelve grams a day is what a monkey will eat in its native environment. So 12 grams a day is really what I believe nature intended for us to have. That pulls a lot of toxins out of the body. Some cancer patients would take 50 grams of vitamin C a day before having any loose stool at all. It all was being used to tie up the toxins."

Diabetes

Recent information suggests, says Dr. Philpott, that diabetes starts with a food allergy and becomes an autoimmune disease. Milk is usually the biggest problem. Many children have an autoimmune reaction in the pancreas, where the antibodies are actually destroying the islet cells.

The later, adult-onset-type diabetes is also related to food allergy, he says, but not one that includes an autoimmune reaction. It is of the IgG type, which causes swelling of the cells so that insulin cannot do its job. "If enough cells become swollen from a food reaction, you simply don't have the blood sugar going from the blood into the cells because too many of them are swollen. If you stop eating the food you're reacting to, the cells won't be swollen and you won't have the diabetes anymore. I have an article called 'Diabetes, A Reversible Disease,' which, along with my *Health Strategies* book, will tell you how to do food testing.

"When I was 54 years old I discovered that I had diabetes. I had painful elbows and bursitis. Milk caused my bursitis, arthritis, and tenosynovitis, and wheat caused my diabetes. That was 20 years ago. I am now 74 and I don't have these ailments anymore. I haven't had them for all of these 20 years because I went on a rotation diet. I had used these methods to help my diabetic patients, but I had no idea that I had a similar need myself until I got dizzy one day. I tested myself for food allergies. I'm thankful that I had learned to help my patients with this because I was able to help myself as well. I rotate my foods and make sure I'm well nourished. I'm in great shape now, whereas I was falling apart at 54."

Detoxifying Your Environment

Dr. Philpott likes his patients to get a good idea of what is going on in their bodies, and in their home and work environments as well. He says that while most people seem to believe their home is a safe haven, the average home is, in fact, very toxic. "There is a serious threat from tap water, for example, and from inhaled substances such as pollen, mold, dust and chemicals that may be in the furniture and the rugs." this is true of the workplace as well, Dr. Philpott says. "Recently we've been hearing about 'sick building syndrome' and how it contributes to disease. That's why I feel it is so important to educate my patients about the reality of their situation and to make them aware of what they can do about it.

"I begin by urging my patients to have an appropriate blood test to see what their vitamin and mineral levels are, and to find out how well they're absorbing and digesting them. A person may be on a good diet and getting the best nutrients but still not be absorbing nutrients adequately. The nutrients may not be going from the gut into the bloodstream and the person may not be getting real benefit from the diet. And nutrient deficiencies are associated with an increased risk of heart disease and cancer."

What follows are some specific suggestions Dr. Philpott makes for detoxification and rebuilding:

Vitamin C. This is probably one of the greatest of the antioxidants and detoxifying substances. It is highly effective at stopping free-radical damage to your tissues because it helps prevent lipid peroxidation at the cellular level. Vitamin C, as do other antioxidants, stops free radicals from destroying the lipid membrane. If you imagine that a body cell is a box, then the walls of that box are made up of lipids and fats. If free radicals repeatedly bombard the fat layer of that cell, sooner or later that box or cell will have a little hole in it. All the substances inside the cell—the mitochondria, proteins, RNA and DNA—will leak out.

Other nutrients. Beyond vitamin C, you need to incorporate selenium, zinc, a good complement of B complex vitamins and vitamins A and E, and beta carotene. Glutathione is a free-radical scavenger and a T-cell stimulant, and thus may help to enhance T-cell function. Incorporating glutathione or N-acetyl-cysteine will improve your ability to fight off infections such as viruses.

Intravenous vitamins. This is one of the best ways to get nutrients from vitamins, says Dr. Philpott. Most people do not have 100 percent absorption using an intramuscular technique, but the intravenous method is by far the best.

Water. Be sure to drink bottled water that is free of metals, bacteria and viral contaminants. "I had one interesting case involving a gentleman from Georgia," relates Dr. Philpott. "He had become ill and was getting worse and worse. He was losing weight and had a whole series of chronic problems. We traced the problem to the water he drank, which came from a well on his property. The well was tested and found to be contaminated with all sorts of metals, as well as bacterial and viral particles. This gentleman was diagnosed as having full-blown AIDS symptoms without ever being positive for HIV. This is an example of how devastating toxic water ingestion can be."

Diet. Minimize red meat in the diet because fats from animals can generate free radicals, which, in turn, can increase lipid peroxidation and increase toxicity in the body. Eat more of a vegetarian diet using organic vegetables.

Exercise. Another way to detoxify is through exercise. A lot of people do not exercise enough or they exercise improperly. Some people feel they're supposed to exercise stringently and become "weekend warriors." They are too tired to work out during the week after work, so once or twice on the weekend they go to the gym. They do too much too soon and may cause themselves damage. They don't get the benefits they expect, and then they drop their program.

Ideally, the body needs to exercise in a routine fashion. It needs at least a half hour's worth of an aerobic activity, one that is nonstop. Most men and women need to do a straight half hour of an activity such as walking, biking or swimming so that the body gets a lot of oxygen and can circulate nutrients to all the tissues. Aerobic exercise will help to rake up the end products of metabolism and push them out of the body. It also pumps lymph fluid around the lymph nodes and channels and throws out particles from the tissues.

Health Begins At Home

Dr. Philpott says that people are becoming more educated about potential problems at home. They are fumigating their rugs, for example, to avoid breathing in the zillions of particles that get into them. Other things that you can do at home to detoxify your environment: Have your water, air and soil tested. Many people now plant their own gardens, but if there are contaminants in the soil, then they are just eating more contaminants. Dr. Philpott also recommends using air purifiers to trap pollen, dust, molds and all sorts of substances that circulate around the house and may be in the rugs, mattresses and furniture. Using filters at home is also a good idea. And mattress and pillow covers will act as barriers; when you're lying in bed you won't be breathing in dust mites that increase your allergy load.

Body Mechanisms Interrelated

"The majority of people believe their symptoms have one or two basic causes," Dr. Philpott says. "They may come to see me with a slight yeast problem, for example, or with slight fatigue or an occasional sore throat. I try to make them realize that there may be five or ten reasons for any one of the problems.

"Let's say someone comes in complaining of frequent tiredness. They may think they have a virus. Perhaps that person was even labeled as having 'chronic fatigue syndrome.' (This is really a poor label because it doesn't describe the cause.) The fatigue might indeed be due to a virus, but they need to look at why the virus is there. The cause may be a defect in immune function and inability to kill a virus, for example. Or it may be due to a nutritional deficiency. The patient may be deficient in zinc or glutathione, which decreases his or her T cells and ability to fight viruses. Or it may be due to a poor diet or a decreased digestion or absorption. The fatigue may also be due to a red blood cell magnesium deficiency. The list goes on and on.

"Instead of looking at one problem by itself, you have to understand that all of the body mechanisms are interrelated. You have to seek secondary and tertiary reasons and causes for problems. The more comprehensive you are, the more likely you will be to solve your problem and regain your health."

Martin Feldman, M.D.
Encouraging Homeostasis

Homeostasis, which is the basis of all life, is a balance between the body's input and output, explains Dr. Feldman. We take in nutrients in the form of calories for energy, and vitamins and minerals for body function. But in addition to this input, the body always has an output of end products that result from its processes. Basically, toxic states are imbalances of the input-output mechanisms. If the output is not clean or efficient, organs, glands or even the cells or body fluids can become congested or suffocated. This means the organs or other functions cannot work properly.

Much has been discussed about the aspects of external toxicity, Dr. Feldman says. "Everybody hears that you breathe in or ingest external toxins. I want to deal with the issue of the internal milieu; from my medical experience, I can share a great deal of information on internal toxic states, and show some of the correlations between symptoms and problems."

He goes on to outline some conditions in which toxicity can be a major cause of the problem:

Allergies. An allergy congesting the body is often a result of toxicity from an input/output problem. Many people have mucus formation as part of an allergy in the throat, nose or sinuses.

Skin problems. One of the skin's functions is to eliminate toxins, and perspiration or sweat is the means through which this normally occurs. Many skin problems arise as a result of toxic overload.

Headaches. Many headache states are triggered by internal toxic reactions.

Immune weakness. Immune problems are often related to an immune toxicity. These problems include frequent colds, lingering colds, repeated viral infections, skin infections, lung problems and bladder problems.

Low energy. Many factors are related to loss of energy, with one aspect being internal toxicity.

Digestive disorders. Many people have inefficient digestive systems. They are not diseased in the classical sense, but the inefficient digestion goes hand in hand with the build-up of toxins.

Obesity. Fat tends to store toxins. So obese people tend to store more toxins in their bodies than do people of normal weight.

Arthritis. There are many causes for arthritis, one being toxicity.

Chemical intolerance. Internal toxicities are commonly related to instances in which a person is intolerant of chemicals, such as perfume.

Food intolerance. People with toxic conditions should reduce congestive foods in their diet. This is simple to do and can be done without consulting a doctor. Congestive foods tend to include dairy products (which create mucus), fats, meat (which tends to overload the whole system with toxicity), refined foods and the chemicals added to food.

The Digestive System

Faulty digestive functioning, Dr. Feldman explains, is often responsible for a loss of homeostasis and resultant toxicity. There are many steps to digestion, and any one of them can be problematic. First, food enters the stomach, where it needs to be efficiently metabolized through the stomach's powerful acid. But stomach acid is commonly inefficient. Next, food goes to the duodenum, where pancreatic enzymes enter the picture. These enzymes may also be out of balance, insufficient, produced incorrectly or their timing may be poor.

In the next stage, the food enters the small intestine, whose job it is to absorb nutrients. The small intestine can also have poor absorption, especially if the friendly bacteria of the small intestine have been pushed out by candida or yeast overgrowth. After leaving the small intestine the food goes through the ileocecal valve and through the colon. So all of these various sites should be looked at to see if they are in a state of homeostasis or if they are causing toxic build-up.

Colon. The colon should be checked first in a toxic analysis because it's a waste generator. "It's the garbage disposal system of the body," Dr. Feldman says. The colon has three parts. It starts at the lower right abdomen near the right hip and ascends along the right side (ascending colon). Then it goes across the mid-abdomen (transverse colon) and then down the left side (descending colon) and into the rectum.

How do you know if your colon is off balance? The first sign to consider, says Dr. Feldman, is discomfort in the lower abdomen. If your discomfort is high up under the sternum where the ribs end, the problem usually involves the stomach or the pancreas. On the other hand, constipation or diarrhea tend to signal a colon problem. Another way to analyze the symptoms is to note if you have a lot of gas. If your food is being metabolized efficiently and cleanly, you won't get a lot of toxic waste products from food and you won't get a lot of fermented gas. Gas is a result of fermented food in the colon that is not metabolized cleanly above.

Cramps tend to reflect an irritable colon. The cramps may appear in the lower abdomen, the right or left side, or over the entire abdomen. Whatever the situation, they are the result of poor colon function and a potential build-up of toxins. One can also examine the stool, which is a very good indicator of the colon's efficiency. If it is well formed with no mucus or undigested matter, and is not loose or hard, you are probably in good health. If your stool is variable from day to day, then the colon might be off the beam.

Irritation of the mucosal lining is common. It's called irritable bowel syndrome, or colitis. One of the many sources of irritation to the colon is food to which a person is intolerant or allergic. "If you test the three parts of the colon you'll see a pattern. When the descending colon alone is irritated—but the ascending and transverse are in good balance and are not irritated—the cause is almost always from intolerance to substances entering through the mouth. Conversely, if the ascending colon is the most severely off balance, that's more an issue of the ecology of that area. The ascending colon is really a fermenting factory. That's where one needs to get the bifidobacterium straight and to feed the friendly bacteria. A yeast overgrowth in that area would also need to be dealt with.

"Some of the ways a person creates a toxic intestine are by eating dairy, sugars, meats and processed foods year in and year out. Exogenous irritants can create a disharmonious intestine. Some safe and excellent sources for reducing or removing the source of that irritation are aloe vera, chlorophyll and slippery elm bark."

Another problem with the colon is an inadequate fluid intake, Dr. Feldman goes on. Many people don't get enough fluid and, as a result, their whole digestive system tends not to flow properly.

Parasites can also cause colon problems. Probably most people on the planet have parasites. The body and the parasites tend to create a symbiotic relationship, whereby the host tolerates the parasites. The parasite doesn't destroy the host totally, and therefore they both can live. We now have excellent non-drug anti-parasite nutrients available. The best is probably grapefruit seed or citrus seed extract. Other good anti-parasitic remedies include black walnut, garlic and, in some cases, artemisia combined with goldenseal.

If you want to restore homeostasis to your colon, here are some of the things Dr. Feldman suggests you consider:

Fiber. One of the first things to look at is the amount of fiber in your diet. Fiber is an essential aspect of the whole digestive process, and is especially important for the colon. There are two kinds of fiber: insoluble and soluble. Insoluble fiber tends to have a mechanical scrubbing or cleansing action. It also forms the stool. Just as important, if not more so, is the soluble fiber, because it helps friendly bacteria. The colon and the small intestine, to some extent, have a biosphere of friendly yeasts as well as all kinds of potentially unfriendly bacteria such as Candida albicans. Part of total body health involves feeding the friendly bacteria. They produce nutrients and keep the whole body in homeostasis by controlling the unfriendly bacteria. If the body is in homeostasis it will keep the unfriendly ones in check.

The best soluble fiber for helping bacteria is pectin. Apples and chia seeds contain a lot of pectin, which is a gelatinous fiber very rich in nutrients. Southwest American Indians, such as the Apaches, used to carry lots of chia seeds on their journeys. They would keep the seeds in their mouths and their saliva would create a gel that gave them much fiber and energy. Glucomannan is another excellent fiber source.

Friendly bacteria. Dr. Feldman mentions a new idea in complementary medicine called the fructo-oligo-saccharides. "These carbohydrates are helpful in encouraging friendly bacteria to be strong and to be in good balance in the colon," he explains.

"Many types of friendly bacteria are also available in health food stores. But most people don't realize that there are differences between them. The colon bacteria are the bifidobacterium bifidum. The small intestine, on the other hand, uses lactobacillus acidophilus. Most people tend to take acidophilus, which is good for the small intestine. They don't usually know to take the bifido part, which is for the colon. There is crossover but basically the colon wants the bifido, not the acidophilus."

Butyric acid. This is especially important to maintain the health of the mucosal lining of the colon and, to some extent, the small intestine. The cells of the inner digestive apparatus are very active. They have a lot of work to do and are in need of really good nutritional support.

Ileocecal valve. The ileocecal valve is located between the ileum, which is the end of the small intestine, and the cecum, which is the beginning of the large intestine. It opens to allow materials to flow through and then closes. It is supposed to keep the flow moving in one direction. The ileocecal valve, however, is often out of balance. It's hard to test for that anatomically, Dr. Feldman says. You have to test it via energy analysis.

"If the valve is not closing well, we have a problem of back flushing where waste material coming out of the small intestine can be flushed backwards. This is a major source of toxic problems. Many people who have back flushing tend to have mucus dripping as part of the problem. The toxic stuff goes into the blood and comes out through the nose.

"There are basically two things you can do for this. Lipid soluble chlorophyll can be taken, as well as a variety of herbal products. You may also need structural help to physically keep that valve closed, and the valve itself could be massaged to help its functioning."

The liver. The liver is well known as a major detoxification organ. It must break down harmful drugs such as medications, alcohol, nicotine and caffeine. To check to see if the liver is working properly and efficiently you can look at your blood liver enzyme levels— the SGOT, SGPT and GGTP. These three readings might be elevated if the liver is inefficient.

One of the problems that can result from a toxic liver is premenstrual syndrome. "The overwhelming majority of women who come to me with moderate or severe PMS have a liver imbalance," Dr. Feldman reports. "Once we get the liver to function optimally, PMS diminishes or disappears." To alleviate some of the symptoms of PMS, he suggests taking gammalinolenic acid (GLA). GLA is found in borage oil, evening primrose oil or black currant seed oil. "You would need to take in the range of 350 mg of the GLA. Also, many women with PMS have low levels of magnesium and need to take a supplement of this mineral. Commonly, there are vitamin B imbalances and an array of other deficiencies as well."

Adult acne can be another liver-related problem. This condition is usually caused by the liver not cleansing the blood properly, says Dr. Feldman, so that the skin becomes the secondary organ of elimination. Other conditions related to liver toxicity can include headaches and hemorrhoids.

To rebalance the liver, the doctor says that it is important to get the digestive apparatus in condition. "First, you need to ask if the digestion system is overloading the liver by inefficient or imperfect digestion. Then check three areas: stomach acid, pancreas enzymes and the small intestine. The small intestine is probably the most complex of the three in terms of correcting, but it is the least commonly off balance. It tends to balance itself very well with lactobacillus acidophilus.

"Next you need to consider, is it the liver only that is off-balance, or is there a liver-gallbladder interconnection? Approximately 25 percent of the time there is gallbladder involvement; the bile liver system is somehow not quite right.

"An herbal approach can usually be used to correct this problem. A few very good herbs to use—although there are many others— include dandelion, red beet root and peppermint. Milk thistle is a wonderful herb for the liver, with or without the gallbladder involvement. The liver loves to have choline, inositol and methionine in the body. This keeps the liver in good health and prevents it from accumulating fat."

Dr. Feldman mentions glutathione, which is acquired through its precursor, N-acetyl-cysteine (NAC). "In certain severe states, you can consider intravenous glutathione, which the liver really appreciates. This is commonly given with vitamin C. It is a great advance of the complementary concept of nutritional support for that organ."

Allergies

On the subject of allergies, Dr. Feldman reminds us that these produce toxins, such as histamine and various other products. Allergies result from an overactive immune function. Anyone with allergies, especially of the congestive kind, must work on getting their immunity into better balance, he says, going on to mention a few things that you can do on your own to this end.

One is to reduce exposure to allergens. In this technological age we are exposed to more and more allergens, which add stress to the system. Dust, for example, is a major-league stressor and should be reduced by using air purifiers, through good housekeeping and by using fewer or no rugs. Molds should also be eliminated. Food and chemical allergies should be noted and dealt with as well.

Another possibility for dealing with this problem is neutralization therapy. This is a homeopathic concept in which the body is given specific dilutions for each antigen. This results in better homeostasis and less toxic allergy.

Low Immune Function

Low immune function is a condition that contrasts sharply with allergy. With low immune function, Dr. Feldman explains, the immune system is underactive, weak and inefficient. "It does not properly clear out pathogens, which can then cause major-league internal toxicity. In my office I use a phase contrast microscope to check the blood in the live state. I take a drop of blood and observe it to see the blood in live motion. I'm amazed at how many bacteria float around in the blood, especially in persons with reduced immune function. Throughout the body, also, there are potential viruses, parasites and yeast, which the immune system must keep in check."

Autoimmune Toxicity

With this problem, the body is so internally nonhomeostatic that it actually attacks its own tissue. This toxic condition is becoming more and more common. "The traditional community recognizes the concept," Dr. Feldman says. In a disease condition termed Hashimoto's thyroiditis, the body produces internal antibodies that attack the normal thyroid tissue, producing disturbance of thyroid function.

Deficiency States

Dr. Feldman points out that "sometimes a problem may not be due to toxicity; it may be related to a deficiency. This can cause further problems if you think you are toxic and you go on an unsupervised fast, which then makes you even more deficient. That is why it is important to get an analysis to see what is truly going on in your system." One of the problems that can be caused by a deficiency state is tiredness. If your energy is low, the adrenals must be checked. If they are low, along with the thyroid, then the energy problems may be partially toxic but more adrenal/thyroid related. The same is true, says Dr. Feldman, with people who are tired from a lack of B-12 or a lack of B vitamins in general. This, again, may be a deficiency and not a toxicity that is making you tired.

Joint and tissue diseases are another area where deficiencies may play a role. Mineral deficiencies are very common here, especially when the digestion is less than perfect. They can result in various problems. Calcium and magnesium deficiencies tend to lead to arthritis. Patients with arthritis commonly have other deficiencies such as low copper, vitamins A, D, B-3 or niacin. Many other joint or connective-tissue problems involve a deficiency of manganese. Low chromium is a very common problem which leads to hypoglycemic tendencies. Low body zinc is associated with problems of immune function, prostate health and skin integrity.

The Lymphatic System

The lymphatic flow system throughout the body is a key to all detoxification, says Dr. Feldman. To help the lymphatic flow, you can increase your fluid intake, exercise and get massages. "Two approaches that I use are herbal formulas and homeopathic remedies. It's very safe and noninvasive. I believe that the future of detoxification thinking should include a focus on lymphatic flow and drainage."

CHAPTER 12
How To Heal Your Body

When it comes to detoxifying the system from a lifetime of accumulated poisons, we have to be realistic: It's not going to happen overnight. We have to be very careful about programs promising immediate rebalancing using powders and potions, magnets or any particular medical therapy. That is not to suggest that these approaches do not have some benefit when done properly. But the days of going to a Herbert Shelton fasting clinic and fasting for 30 to 40 days until you've either cured or killed yourself are over. We now have to look very carefully at what is occurring in our bodies.

The first thing you must do is get an honest evaluation of what is actually happening inside the blood cells by taking some blood chemistry tests. These tests are generally not expensive and not painful, but they're absolutely necessary. One of the most common tests is a viral titer which measures the immunoglobulin, the serum proteins that include all known antibodies, in blood. The measurement of immunoglobulin-G (IgG) tells if you were at one time infected with a virus or bacteria, while the measurement of immunoglobulin-M (IgM) tells you whether you are currently infected, to what degree you are infected, and what this infection might be doing to your system.

Why are these things important to know? When I began to look at the blood chemistry of people with AIDS and chronic fatigue syndrome, I saw something unusual. With the exception of the HIV virus, the blood chemistries were virtually indistinguishable. They both had varying elevated titers (a measure of the concentration of a virus) of hepatitis A, B or C; mycoplasm; herpes 1, 2 and 6; cytomegalovirus; Epstein-Barr virus; parasites; and syphilis. On a nutritional level, they suffered from malabsorption syndrome, defective pancreas, adrenal exhaustion, underactive thyroid, a deficient thymus gland, and general toxicity of the liver. These maladies are common in people with cancer. In fact, people with AIDS, chronic fatigue syndrome, hepatitis, and cancer, have blood chemistries that are quite similar, with the exception of HIV and specific cancer markers.

My findings raised several puzzling questions. They led me to ask if it was possible that what we call AIDS and chronic fatigue syndrome were one and the same. Should AIDS really be diagnosed as chronic fatigue syndrome? Also, by treating AIDS with toxic drugs, are we only further exacerbating the condition and creating a whole generation of iatrogenic (treatment-induced) disease, in which the treatment becomes worse than the condition? What would happen if we reversed that condition by first cleansing the body of these obvious cofactors contributing to the destruction of the immune system and then building up the immune system without overstimulating it, thereby preventing a hypervigilant immune reaction leading to autoimmune disease?

This theory proved to be absolutely correct. A group of physicians used one of three treatment modalities with their AIDS and chronic fatigue patients. One modality was a detoxification, cleansing and rebuilding program using such methods as IV drips of vitamin C, glutathione, inositol, cysteine and licorice extract, and orally or rectally administered bitter melon. This treatment worked extremely well in helping people recover to a point where they were functioning even more healthfully than they had been before they contracted these diseases.

The other group was given the same protocol but was not detoxed. They weren't told to stop any of their negative habits. They continued to drink their four to 10 cups of coffee a day, eat sugar, smoke, eat saturated fats, and take other medications such as antibiotics. They made modest, though not overwhelming, gains, but they still did not have the same incidence of full-blown AIDS.

Those in the group who had chronic fatigue syndrome didn't lapse into becoming completely debilitated.

A third protocol was established whereby patients were encouraged to exercise and foster more positive spiritual and emotional attitudes along with their detoxification program. This group did the best of all. Several subjects who went into remission had no HIV active in their bodies at all. Their immune systems became stronger and healthier than before.

While this study was being conducted, I was also training a group of marathoners. I've trained some of the greatest athletes in the world, such as Joan Rollin, Sam Skinner, Queenie Thompson, Franco Pantoni and Thelma Wilson. These people are world champions for their various age groups in running or power walking competitions. They were not lead athletes when they began their program five or six years ago—just normal functioning people. By super-building their immune systems, compensating for the stress of their exercise regimen and coming to understand the importance of stress management, guided visualization and positive affirmation, these people have not only been able to compete and achieve each of their goals, they've sustained their level of competition for years, where most other athletes would have burned out or slipped back.

In the process, another group of athletes was inspired by the example of these individuals and wanted to be trained. I agreed to this, but with the stipulation that I first wanted to know what was going on with their biochemistries so we could quantify baseline levels, measure their blood six months later and then see where they'd gone. I wanted them to keep diaries so that they could see that if they overtrained it was destructive to the system. I told them that unless I missed my guess, they would start to see some dormant viruses become active.

None of these people had any risk factors. They were not sexually promiscuous and a few were even virgins. They did not drink, smoke or take any drugs. Many were vegetarians. You could say this was an exceptional group.

Here's what was interesting: When the blood chemistries came back I was absolutely flabbergasted to see mycoplasm, parasites, and almost all the different viruses with the exception of HIV in all of their blood. Mind you, these are healthy people. These people are the ultimate health enthusiasts, people who have done no harm and have tried to do everything right. Yet they had many of the different viruses that we have been claiming are the causes of different diseases.

Clearly it is not just the viruses in people that cause sickness. Viruses and bacteria, the very substances that can lessen the quality of life and ultimately destroy us, are with us at all times. Based upon this sampling of very healthy people, we can probably assume that about 95 percent of the American population carry most of the different types of viruses, bacteria and parasites to some degree.

Disease As A Gradual Process

What I see happening is, as people age and do not pay attention to their immune systems, as they continue to be exposed to low-level toxicity from such things as pollutants in the air, water and soil, these people—who are not doing anything to actively hurt themselves—in time, have systems that become overwhelmed. Then it's a matter of chance as to what will be the trigger—the emotional crisis, the chronic stress, the lack of exercise, the multiple nutritional deficiencies, the bingeing, the exposure to something toxic in the environment, or combinations of any or all of these— that one day causes their system to no longer be able to maintain homeostasis and to actively start to process disease. At that point, a messenger is triggered within the body to allow what otherwise were nonpathogenic viruses and bacteria to become more pathogenic and more viral. Hence, symptoms, which become the healing crisis of the body, begin to appear.

By the time we actually see the result of a tumor or asthma or some other condition, it's actually the end stage of the disease process, not the beginning, contrary to medical dogma. It may have taken 10, 20 or 30 years to hurt the system, but surely, any system not vigorously protected and fortified does fail. Therefore the idea that we are either healthy because we have no symptoms of disease, or sick when we get a symptom, is so foolish as to be virtually useless as a guide.

Generally, disease or health doesn't just happen. At any given time we are actively processing wellness or disease by what we inadvertently or intentionally feed our body, mind and spirit. Some people rationalize about needing their job, even though it makes them sick, so they continue to work in a stressful or toxic environment, thinking their economic salvation is more important than their physical and emotional health. As long as they don't have a disease, they speculate that maybe it won't happen to them. But that's like the smokers who figure that as long as there is no cancer on their lungs maybe it's not going to happen to them. In both cases they're playing a game of Russian roulette in which they eventually run out of empty chambers. Sooner or later the body is going to be affected.

You need to understand right up front that "disease" and "wellness" are not isolated states but part of an ongoing process. All the hazards I've outlined in this book—background radiation, sleeping next to a digital clock, sitting too close to a television, working too close to a computer, drinking chlorinated water, having mercury fillings, getting too many dental X-rays, taking antibiotics too often, eating excess sugar, eating red meat and saturated fats, breathing in formaldehyde and asbestos, etc.—add to the process of disease, often without your being consciously aware of it. And remember that the body cannot differentiate between an intentional assault and an unintentional one. Every negative thing you do adds one more element to that disease process.

It is important to remember, too, that emotional assaults, as well as physical ones, take their toll. If you get angry and impatient because traffic is tied up, for example, your adrenals oversecrete adrenaline because your body is exhibiting a fight-or-flight response. That reaction served a purpose in ancient times when man needed to react to life-threatening situations in order to survive. While the fight-or-flight response sometimes has a place in today's world, overall it does more harm than good. In most of the emotionally stressful situations we encounter today, the fight-or-flight reflex is useless. Yet it's hard to just turn it off. Your body often still perceives situations as life-threatening, and so it secretes too much adrenaline. That reaction kills you bit by bit.

The immune system makes constant adaptations and adjustments to protect you, to try to rejuvenate your system and to try to defend you by working to encapsulate foreign agents 24 hours a day. People with absolutely cavalier attitudes operate under the foolish assumption that unless something they ingest immediately causes them to drop dead, they can safely eat, drink or breathe anything. These people often end up with diabetes, arthritis, congestive heart failure, colon cancer or breast cancer, and then wonder, Why me?

Medicine is neither in the business of creating a wellness model, nor is it really preventive. It deals instead with pathology. And it hasn't even been able to be objective in understanding what causes disease, because it looks for single causes. This brings in the economic side of medicine, as embodied by the simplistic concept of the single cure. While the single cure may be good for business, it has nothing to do with prevention or effective nontoxic treatment. When you look at it from that perspective you can understand why we have nothing resembling progress to show for the $1.2 trillion spent in 1994 on sickness care. Cancer, heart disease, diabetes, arthritis, obesity, mental illness and AIDS, for example, are on the rise. If our current model worked, we'd see a concomitant decrease in disease. Obviously, the only model we can trust is one in which we place first and foremost the creative and constructive realignment of our lifestyle in order to optimize our wellness.

The Path To Wellness

Getting Tested

When it comes to selecting a program, you first must understand what is going on in your system. And to get a handle on your system, you have to get some tests done. These tests will allow you to understand what you need to do in order to cleanse properly. You can have allergy tests done, for example, to determine whether or not your fatigue, candida, PMS, migraine, insomnia, or other symptoms are due to your having chemical or food sensitivities or to anything unhealthy in your environment or diet. You can do these with your regular physician or with a physician who uses applied kinesiology, which is testing the energy systems of the body to tell you if something is positive and strengthening or negative and weakening. You can see this when someone who is allergic or chemically sensitive is given a grain of sugar under the tongue; it weakens that person immediately. When they're given vitamin C it can strengthen them immediately.

Another important test to get done is the viral panel mentioned earlier in the chapter. Also get a test to determine the amount of heavy metals in your body. These tests can determine if enzyme systems are being adversely affected by lead, cadmium, mercury or other metals. You can also get tested to see if your silver amalgam fillings are outgassing mercury from your teeth. Often these need to be removed and replaced with less toxic materials.

Take a glucose tolerance test (GTT) to measure blood levels of glucose, which is the sugar that the body uses. Glucose is usually maintained at a constant level by means of insulin and other hormones, but there are certain imbalanced states in which the glucose level is too high or too low. These can cause you to feel lethargic, dizzy and irritable. The GTT, a simple, inexpensive test, can determine if you have blood sugar imbalances that would precipitate these mood and energy fluctuations.

You can also get a classic blood test (SMA-24), which will give you a lot of information with which to work. It will let you know, for example, whether you're too acid or too alkaline, and whether your uric acid, calcium and cholesterol levels are in balance.

You should also get an impedance test. This simple test involves clamping an electrode onto your large toe and running a painless current through the body for about two seconds to determine your percentage of body fat, lean muscle tissue and water. Healthy men should be between 18 and 21 percent fat; women should be around 23 percent fat. Most people, however, are 5 to 10 points above that. This test can tell you if you are overfat even if you seem skinny. Ideally, you want more lean muscle and less fat, to help your arteries and your body overall.

Once you've gotten your tests done, at least you know what conditions you're working with. Now you're ready to start a cleansing and rebuilding program. What are the various therapies that can make a difference? Let's say your tests come back showing that you've got clogged arteries. You can begin by getting a proper nutritional program for that. Dr. Dean Ornish has shown that a group of patients made significant progress in reversing their atherosclerosis after a year of eating a vegetarian diet that had only 10 to 15 percent fat, in combination with exercise and a stress management program. You could also look at chelation therapy, along with other healing modalities.

Choosing A Therapy

Chelation Therapy

Traditionally, people have been led to believe that there is no way of really helping the heart. You simply have to take your medications and accept your condition or undergo risky bypass operations, which offer no hope of lasting change. Fortunately, there is an alternative. Hundreds of thousands of people have undergone chelation treatments for circulatory problems, with a great many having lasting success. Many heart patients who were not expected to live are fully alive today and leading normal, healthy and productive lives. One such patient, for example, reported to me on my radio program that after he'd had three bypass operations, his cardiologist had given up on him. His cardiologist told him to have a heart transplant, and when he said he would not hear of it, the doctor just told him to go home and get his affairs in order. Fortunately, he found chelation therapy, and he reports that now, "I do not take even one heart pill and I have never been in the hospital since. I'm feeling better than ever and able to work between 12 and 15 hours a day and to travel over 80,000 miles a year for my business."

How chelation works. The term chelation is derived from the Greek root "chele," meaning claw. It refers to a molecule that is able to grab onto, deactivate and remove a mineral from the body. The process involves the infusion of the amino acid EDTA into the bloodstream, which moves through the blood vessels and removes excesses of iron, copper, lead and various other metals that are implicated in disease. It also decreases the calcium and helps solidify plaque in our vessels. As the plaque is reduced, and through a variety of other biochemical mechanisms, blood flow all over the body improves. In addition, chelation provides greater antioxidant activity, minimizing the free-radical damage to our cells and tissues.

When combined with a change in lifestyle, this treatment may benefit people in a variety of ways. It may slow down or reverse the aging process by keeping free radicals in check. It can also strengthen oxidation to the heart and blood vessels, thereby helping major organs to revitalize. In addition, it can help reverse many other disease processes, such as strokes, Alzheimer's disease, diabetes, intermittent claudication (leg cramps) and poor circulation; and eliminate heavy metals such as lead, mercury and cadmium, which poison the body. In contrast to most conventional treatments, which address symptoms only, chelation therapy treats the basic causes of underlying illness, thereby reversing the disease process and restoring health.

As to precisely how chelation works, we know that EDTA removes metals and that it's not metabolized in the body at all. It just comes in, grabs a mineral and goes out through the urine. In so doing it brings about a number of profound reactions in the body, which result in therapeutic effects. For example, as people age and as disease occurs we get an accumulation of calcium in and around the cells of the soft tissues. Yes, we do like calcium, but we don't like it in our arteries or our joints. The EDTA helps remove this excessive calcium from the wrong places. And EDTA helps to stop excessive free-radical formation, which results in destruction of cell membranes and serves as a common pathway for diseases such as multiple sclerosis, cancer, arterialsclerosis, and so on. So EDTA does a number of remarkable things in the body.

Eliminating several heart problems. If you understand something about the role of the heart in the circulatory system then you'll understand how chelation helps. Basically, the heart is a pump composed of four chambers working through a contraction of the muscles. Blood enters the right side of the heart and is then contracted to both lungs where it picks up oxygen. It then returns to the left chambers of the heart and is pumped out by the left ventricle into the arteries in order to deliver oxygenated blood to all the tissues of the body. After passing through the tissues, blood returns to the heart through the veins and the process repeats itself.

When the coronary arteries become clogged because of atherosclerosis, a hardening of the arteries, the circulation going to the heart is impaired. This functioning is detrimental because the heart muscle needs oxygen and nutrients from the blood in order to contract properly. Therefore, when the circulation of blood is impaired, the function of the heart is damaged as well. The heart may then have problems with electrical conductivity, which could result in abnormal heart rhythms. As arterialsclerosis continues and damages vessels in the body, all of our tissues suffer. Remember, our blood carries numerous essential substances to cells of all types.

Another factor important for normal beating of the heart is magnesium. A lack of magnesium may cause the aorta or the coronary blood vessels to go into spasm. This, in turn, causes poor functioning because it reduces the amount of blood to the heart muscles. Poor or uncoordinated muscle contraction can cause elevated blood pressure. And when oxygen delivery to the heart is poor, the body can receive signals from the heart in the form of pain called angina. Magnesium is added to the chelation treatment to help relax muscles so more blood can flow through them. It also helps improve blood pressure.

Quite often the degree of arterial disease present is incorrectly estimated by taking an oversimplified or overly mechanical approach to the problem. The damage is simply judged by the size of the blockage in the arteries. In other words, if the blockage is big, then it is said that you have severe problems with circulation, and if it is moderate or if no blockage is seen, you are usually given the impression that no circulatory disease exists whatsoever. But this is not necessarily true. It's important to realize that the arteries are more than pipes delivering fuel to the body. The arteries are living structures. Their linings have about 98 different enzymatic systems whose purpose is not only to prevent blockage build-up damage but to allow oxygen and nutrients to permeate freely through them into the heart muscle and other tissues.

It's been found that in circulatory disease, usually 46 out of these 98 enzymatic systems are destroyed or limited. This leads to the deposition of heavy metals and calcium, and free-radical pathology, which further leads to the formation of insoluble complexes being deposited into the intima, or the inner lining of the arteries. These insoluble complexes bind the lipids of the outer membrane of the arterial walls, which leads to increased collagen, a scar tissue, which prevents oxygen and nutrients from permeating the lining freely. This destroys the integrity of normal circulatory physiology since the final objective of this arterial supply system is getting oxygen to the cells.

If nutrients and oxygen are not delivered to the heart muscle, it will begin to degenerate. First the metabolism of the heart muscle cells will switch from aerobic (with oxygen) to anaerobic (without oxygen). The body uses this as a back-up system to try to preserve the function of the cells. But this eventually leads to a build-up of acid between the cells in the interstitial spaces. In the long run, cells devoid of oxygen become exposed to free-radical activity, which causes them to weaken and die. Very often accompanying this process is an increase in nerve sensitivity, and the person experiences the pain of angina.

In the early stages of this pathology, in which the permeability of the oxygen is impaired, you may have classical angina symptoms, suggesting blockages in the arteries. Yet you may have normal angiographic studies; in other words, no coronary artery blockages are seen on the angiogram. At this point you are usually told that no circulatory disease exists. It is here that I believe that chelation should be used as a preventive measure before heart disease becomes evident. I think anyone over the age of 30 should be getting chelation therapy. It's the most effective rejuvenating and detoxifying system there is.

There's yet another aspect to this. Because the number one killer in this country is heart disease, and because more people suffer from heart disease—including hypertension, clogged arteries and arterialsclerosis—than from any other condition, chelation therapy helps the heart in a number of ways. For instance, it cleanses the body of toxic material such as heavy metals and moves calcium out of soft tissues so that normal contractions can resume. When you heal the internal body the calcium goes to the site of an injury and acts like an internal scab. After you heal, the calcium goes away, but if you keep on injuring yourself, for example with daily cigarette smoking or drinking, the calcium builds up and arterialsclerosis forms around it. EDTA chelation can go in and remove that calcium. When accompanied by a change in lifestyle, it can reverse some of the effects of constant, continued injury.

Many doctors I know around the country are using chelation therapy in heart treatment with great success. One such doctor is Kirk Morgan, director of the Morgan Medical Clinic and Assistant Clinical Professor at the University of Louisville in Kentucky, who has been using chelation successfully on heart patients since 1982 with 90 percent or better improvement in people with hardening of the arteries. In his recently published article, "Myocardial Ischemia Treated with Nutrients in Intravenous EDTA Chelation," Dr. Morgan documented the results of two patients with exercise-induced angina pectoris who were treated with chelation. After fewer than 40 treatments, electrocardiographic heart tracings (EKG's) of these patients showed abnormalities becoming normal on repeat stress testing 15 months after beginning treatment. Both patients demonstrated total cessation of all symptoms. In addition, their defective kidney function returned to normal.

Most other studies in this area show equally dramatic results. Dr. Albert Scarchilli of Farmington Hills, Illinois, was involved in a retrospective study of more than 19,000 cases of patients with peripheral vascular disease. It was revealed by thermoscan that 97 percent of those who received chelation therapy showed significant improvement. And Dr. Michael Jansen of Cambridge, Massachusetts, showed that his patients' angina pain was relieved in 97 percent of cases after chelation therapy. In all, approximately 4,000 scientific articles have been written on various aspects of the process.

Remember that the number of infusions will vary from patient to patient. And generally a whole program goes along with it.

Removing heavy metals. Heavy metal toxicity is a growing problem in the United States. We live in an environment that's polluted, and this pollution gets into our food and drinking water. Additionally, if the air you are breathing contains any metal, you'll pick that right up. The average person right now has a body burden of lead that is a thousand times greater than people had just 500 years ago. We're all, to some extent, lead poisoned, some much worse than others.

Chelation therapy is approved for the removal of these heavy metals. However, mainstream medicine would prefer not to see it used except when levels in the body are very, very high. The problem with this thinking is that since toxic substances like lead are dangerous and have no biological function, they don't belong in the body at all and should be removed at any level.

Unfortunately, heavy metals do not show their tremendous burden to the body until a great deal of harm has already been done. Only when damage is in its acute phase will symptoms like headaches and dizziness appear. But when chelation therapy is used it usually lowers the level of toxic metals in the body significantly in only 5 or 10 treatments.

Osteoporosis and blood pressure. EDTA also acts as a calcium binder. As serum calcium decreases, the body responds by secreting parathyroid hormone, which helps mobilize calcium from abnormal tissue sites and move it into bones where it's needed. In this way, chelation is an indirect treatment for osteoporosis. In addition, with EDTA acting as a calcium chelator, the blood pressure may go down 10 to 20 points and high blood pressure medications may become less needed or altogether unnecessary.

Other benefits. Chelation can benefit the entire circulatory system. You often have atherosclerotic plaque of the little vessels of the kidneys even before the heart is affected, and this weakens the body's cleansing process. By regulating the amount of EDTA accordingly and adding vitamin C to repair the tissues, the little vessels of the kidneys will get cleaned out. Then we can increase the amount of EDTA and ultimately clean the whole vascular system: the heart, kidneys, liver, pancreas and brain.

Chelation is especially helpful to diabetics. Diabetes generally involves the arteries. The blood sugar simply happens to be an indicator of how rapidly the disease is progressing. Chelation will open up insulin receptors and may decrease the body's need for extra insulin.

In addition, chelation improves circulation to the brain and may prevent the onset of a stroke or aid in alleviating the effects of one. A large study indicates that an imbalance of facial circulation is indicative of people prone to have strokes. Chelation softens the arteries in the neck and brain and improves the blood flow, resulting in abnormal thermography scans (infrared scans of the head and feet) returning to normal.

Some people with Alzheimer's disease also benefit from this therapy. They function much better, are more alert and are able to fit into their family setting more appropriately than before treatment. In people who succumb to this disease, delicate nerve tendrils, which are responsible for allowing one part of the brain to talk to another, short out, which results in a loss of short-term memory. When chelation therapy is given, things change. One study on the effects of chelation on the brain was performed by Dr. Edward McDonough. In that test, an independent psychologist tested 35 people with a battery of psychological tests prior to 30 treatments of EDTA chelation and 20 treatments of hyperbaric oxygen, which were given concurrently. When retested, every person showed I.Q. improvement.

Tens of thousands of people have also been successfully treated with chelation for intermittent claudication, a type of peripheral vascular disease involving poor circulation in the legs that may produce pain in the calf muscles upon walking. Dramatic results showed sores and ulcers that had not healed for a year disappeared after chelation therapy.

Gangrene responds as well. Over the years, people who were supposed to have had their legs amputated improved days after treatment. Some of these people are now walking on their own legs.

Another disease that responds well to chelation is macular degeneration, a disease of the eye that causes blindness. Although many ophthalmologists don't believe there is a treatment for this condition, chelation practitioners have found that many macular degeneration patients improved significantly, to the point where those who hadn't been able to read for several years before treatment could now do so.

The treatment has been responsible for the alleviation of numerous other conditions, such as migraine headaches, scleroderma, hypertension, arthritis, impotence, kidney calcification, high cholesterol and multiple sclerosis. So you can see that the detoxification aspects of chelation therapy are quite remarkable. The whole idea is that chelation is the pound of prevention that's worth a hundred pounds of cure. It's been proven effective as a means of helping detoxify and then stimulating the immune system.

There are approximately 800 chelating therapists in the United States. You can get the list of these from the American College of the Advancement of Medicine (1-800-532-3688).

Herbs

Herbs are wonderful aids to healing and, when appropriately chosen, are highly beneficial to any detoxification program. There are some general benefits that can be derived from using herbs, and some specific benefits from particular herbs. Any herb that helps improve overall health will assist in the detoxification process. More specifically, though, there are herbs that really focus on each of the primary pathways of elimination in the body. Herbalist David Hoffman, from California, suggests some herbs you might consider using to help revitalize the various systems responsible for cleansing:

Herbs for the liver. A healthy functioning liver is imperative for detoxification. There are herbs called hepatics that stimulate overall liver activity in general, but for detoxification specifically you should consider herbs called antihepatotoxics. It has only recently been discovered that some herbs can protect the liver cells from chemical toxicity as well as help liver cells over time to overcome pre-existing toxicity. They facilitate rejuvenation of a damaged liver and increase resistance to damage from chemical poisons.

Certainly in the Western world the best known of these is milk thistle. Others that do similar work include licorice, and some Chinese herbs, such as bupleurum, Siberian ginseng and schizandra. These herbs, especially milk thistle, are generally safe when used for short periods of time and in small, professionally managed doses, and can be used effectively to reverse a whole range of liver damage and to protect the liver from chemical ruin.

Herbs for the bowels. There are many herbs available that promote bowel movement. You have a choice between those that are mild yet effective and stronger ones that are effective and still safe. There are also very powerful herbs that have long-term toxic problems associated with them. This last group includes herbs such as senna and cascara sagrada, which are widely used in natural foods circles for their laxative effects. Unfortunately, in the long term they also are physically addictive and will usually result in persons not being able to have a bowel movement on their own. Therefore, they are not recommended. Safer herbs include dandelion root and yellow dock, which are also good blood cleansers.

Herbs for the kidneys. Several herbs that support kidney function are available. They range from those that promote diuresis (the excretion of urine), such as dandelion leaf, to those that will soothe inflammation of the urinary tract as well as stimulate secretion. One very good herb for this purpose is corn silk.

Antimicrobial herbs such as bearberry, also known as uva-ursi, may prevent cystitis or other infection in the bladder. Bearberry may also help relieve pain from bladder stones and gravel, and help where bedwetting is a problem.

There are stronger herbs that, again, should be avoided, such as juniper and other herbs with strong, irritating oils. They do work well but in the long term will have toxic contraindications for people with weak kidneys.

Herbs for the skin. The skin, as the largest detoxification organ of the body, may need special attention if it is to work optimally. All the herbs known as "alterative" and "diaphoretic" will help the skin. Those to keep in mind include nettles, cleavers and burdock; there are many more as well.

Herbs for the lungs. Herbs to consider here vary, depending upon whether you have been a smoker or not. If you have smoked, the appropriate herb to support the lungs in its detoxification work would be elecampane. Taken as a tea, elecampane has been known to quiet a cough and to help overcome respiratory problems. The nonsmoker should consider something less strong, such as mullein. For nasal congestion or other respiratory ailments you can try adding a handful of mullein flowers to hot water and breathing in the vapors.

Herbs for the immune system. Supporting the body's immune system gives you better ability to cope with stress and is important in preventing disease. According to Rob McCaleb, president of the nonprofit Herbal Research Foundation and an adviser to the Department of Health and Human Services' newly established Office of Alternative Medicine, adaptogenic herbs, such as Siberian ginseng, help us by supporting the immune system and making our natural disease-fighting cells stronger and more active. Adaptogenic substances, by the way, don't just serve one specific function. They can help the body adapt to different needs at different times.

Astragalus, another immunomodulating herb, is being closely looked at for its potential benefits to cancer and AIDS patients. In one study performed at the University of Texas, for example, astragalus was shown to completely restore the immune function of cells taken from cancer patients. Astragalus is especially effective when combined with legustrum.

Another good herb to keep on hand for boosting the immune system at the onset of a cold or flu is echinacea. This native American herb could also be considered for alleviating conditions arising from contaminated blood, such as eczema, acne and boils.

Anti-viral herbs. Certain herbs are noted for their anti-viral activity, and you may want to include them in a cleansing/rebuilding program. These include garlic, echinacea, goldenseal, and St. Johnswort. Goldenseal is especially effective when combined with myrrh. Both goldenseal and St. Johnswort, however, should be used on a temporary basis only, as they are medicinal and can produce negative effects in the long term. Garlic, on the other hand, should be taken every day.

Bio-Oxidative Therapies

If you are beset by viruses, bacteria, parasites and a defective immune system, as your starting point for a cleansing program you should consider a professionally supervised nutritional program accompanied by different therapies in the bio-oxidative category. This could include ozone therapy, which is generally a way of killing viruses, bacteria or microbes. This therapy is done by pumping ozone (O_3) into the body through the rectum or by the withdrawal of a half pint of blood from the arm, infusing it with ozone until it turns bright red, and then fusing it back. These methods are very effective but should only be done under medical supervision.

How bio-oxidative therapy can improve health. Dr. Charles Farr, of Oklahoma City, Oklahoma, a biochemist and board-certified physician, is greatly enthusiastic about bio-oxidative medicine's potential: "There has never been anything to come along more effective than bio-oxidation," says Dr. Farr. "I've seen people come in wheelchairs and go out walking." He goes on to explain how bio-oxidative medicine can help improve a person's health: "Bio-oxidative medicine simply describes a living process of the body that comes about through oxidative chemistry. The people doing oxidative therapies are most interested in ways of modifying or reversing the effects of damage that occurs when the body reduces oxidative reactions. When you reduce oxidative reactions, it's like putting your life out a piece at a time. Our purpose is to try to lessen that process.

"We use things like hydrogen peroxide, ozone and vitamin C. We also use what are normally called antioxidants. Whether you give a person ascorbic acid or ozone, the end result is basically the same: A transfer of electrons occurs. Large amounts of vitamin C also increase the production of hydrogen peroxide in the body and make it available for whatever the body needs. By using hydrogen peroxide by itself, you're just adding to what's already there. Using ozone, you're also converting that to hydrogen peroxide and adding to what's there." Dr. Farr says that when you use these tools to try to improve the oxidative rate, all functions of the body, including immune responses, come back to life.

Ed McCabe, a Syracuse, New York journalist and author of the bestselling book *Oxygen Therapies*, notes that another important function of oxygen therapy is its ability to kill pathogens. Says McCabe, "The basic idea is that 90 percent of the bacteria, viruses, fungi and pathogens that cause all disease are anaerobic. That means they can't live in the presence of oxygen. The reason everyone is diseased is because fluids in the body are full of all these microbes which are alive and replicating within the blood, plasma and cells. If the body fluids get enough oxygen—and remember that we are two-thirds water, so that means we're going to have to repeatedly use a good quantity of the active forms of oxygen to clean out 100 or more pounds of fluid—the oxygen oxidizes or burns up all the offending bacteria, viruses, funguses and pathogens. People flood their bodies with oxygen and at that point it cleans their bodies up and eliminates the pathogenic—or bad— bacteria, viruses and fungi."

Oxygen therapy can be of benefit to anyone. McCabe points out, "It is an excellent preventative because if you have enough oxygen in your body, when the virus or bacteria tries to invade your body and cause you harm, it's burnt up by the oxygen. It's great if you're just coming down with a disease because the added oxygen makes it real easy for you to turn your condition around since you're in the initial stages. If you're seriously ill with a chronic, long-term illness, the therapy takes longer, naturally, but we've seen amazing turn-arounds even in, for example, AIDS patients with no T cells. They'll get oxygen therapy once a week and improve their level of health to the point of becoming perfectly healthy. In essence, they're replacing their own immune system, which isn't functioning, with an external immune system, and the external immune system is ozone therapy.

McCabe continues, "I personally have known about a dozen people—I've seen their medical records—who have gone from being HIV positive to HIV negative. Some people have used the over-the-counter methods of oxygen therapy which is a more long-term process for getting rid of all the secondary diseases. They get completely healthy yet still test positively for the HIV virus. But we don't really know if that means much because no one has ever proven the HIV virus causes AIDS."

Dr. Kirk Morgan of Prospect, Kentucky, studied hydrogen peroxide therapy on a large group of people with a variety of ailments and found most subjects to have a highly positive response to treatment. His findings, which were published in the *Townsend Newsletter for Doctors*, reflected statistically impressive success rates for intravenous hydrogen peroxide infusions in the treatment of peripheral vascular disease, pulmonary disease, viral illness, bronchitis, chronic fatigue syndrome and Epstein-Barr virus.

Oxygen—the invisible therapy. If oxygen therapies are so tremendously effective, why aren't they being used by most medical practitioners today? One important reason: No drug company will research and fund it. As Dr. Morgan points out, "No drug company is going to spend $50 million to research the effects of hydrogen peroxide in order for the FDA to approve of it since, the next drug company down the street can make that available without spending $50 million." In other words, hydrogen peroxide can't be patented. It is, after all, a byproduct of our metabolism; a great amount is made by our own white blood cells and used to kill germs.

Inherent dangers of oxygen therapy. "Hydrogen peroxide is potent," Dr. Morgan warns. "Too much oxygen can be a problem; retinal fibroplasia, for example, can occur from it." It therefore must be carefully administered by a doctor. He explains that oxygen is like fire. When you give a patient oxygen, oxidation occurs at a higher rate, which is what happens when you have combustion, or fire. Dr. Morgan says, "All fire is not bad, but it is potent. We couldn't make our cars run without it or have industry. It causes a release of energy and we need that."

The amount of hydrogen peroxide given to a patient must be

carefully administered by a physician. Dr. Morgan reports that the concentration given these days by physicians is generally less than the amount used years ago.

He also notes that ozone therapy, which has been available in Europe for 50 years, is more easily tolerated than hydrogen peroxide therapy by most patients. It's given by a direct intravenous infusion or by mixing the blood with it and then giving the blood back to the patient. "It may be a little better for oxidizing germs and abnormal tissue, such as you find in cancer," Dr. Morgan says. "Cancer does very poorly in the presence of oxygen. This was proven by Warburg, who won a Nobel prize in the late 1930s for his work showing cancer not growing in the presence of O_2, just plain oxygen. He sealed cancer cells in jars and pumped oxygen into them. The cancer cultures died because they couldn't survive in the presence of oxygen."

Ed McCabe agrees that "ozone therapy is the best form of bio-oxidative treatment. The standard way of giving it in this country at this point in time is injecting pharmaceutical-grade ozone into the patient's body. Unlike air, which has nitrogen in it, this gas is strictly pure oxygen, so there is no danger of embolism."

Other Healing Modalities

Colonic irrigation. Colonic irrigation is important because the health of the colon is crucial. In beginning a detoxification program you should have one or two irrigations during the first week to start the debris that's in the intestines moving. But also, a diet high in fiber, especially fruit and grain fibers, will facilitate a sweeping of the intestines with generally multiple bowel movements to help cleanse them. Added to that, vitamin C could be taken several times throughout the day to help facilitate this action.

Cleansing foods and juices. The primary diet to consider when cleansing is a sensible one fortifying you with vitamins and minerals to give you lasting energy and to boost your immune system to greater health.

One important food class to consider is sea vegetables, which are rich in calcium, protein and many important trace minerals lacking in our soil today. Foods from the ocean, such as kombu, wakame, hijiki, nori, agar, kuzu, algin, alaria, sea palm and dulce are therefore extremely important to good health and should be eaten at least four times a week. They are rich sources of potassium and iodine, which help nourish the thyroid gland and the central nervous system. Sea vegetables can be used in soups or salads. They are generally prepared by first soaking them for five minutes, rinsing them with cold water, soaking and rinsing them again and then cooking them for about 10 minutes. They can be chilled in the refrigerator and chopped up for salads, or heated and put into hot soups and entrees.

Also be sure to include cruciferous vegetables on a daily basis. Known for their powerful healing benefits, they include broccoli, cauliflower, brussels sprouts and asparagus. Additional healing vegetables include dandelion greens, mustard greens, cabbage, watercress, buckwheat and sunflower sprouts. While all vegetables are good, these are extremely beneficial.

Garlic, which has been used throughout history as the most healing food herb there is overall, should be served at least two to three times a day.

For the digestive system, eat blueberries, strawberries and cinnamon. Papaya also helps with digestion. Pears are a wonderful cleanser, as are prunes, for helping to eliminate constipation. Apples are a wonderful colon cleanser and an overall tonic as well. Also, watermelon is an excellent blood purifier and a natural diuretic.

Eat as many salads as you want. Include sprouts, edible flowers, dark green vegetables and starchy vegetables slightly steamed. You can make a delicious dressing from canola oil, flax seed oil or olive oil and balsamic vinegar, adding different seasonings to make it more tasty.

Raw juices are extremely beneficial to your health. Some that I like include a combination of dandelion, cucumber, kale, arugula, Swiss chard and parsley. Generally use only an ounce of these darker juices and dilute with milder juices and spring water. The milder juices are made from cabbage, apple, beet, carrot, celery and cucumber. You can also try wheat grass for its cleansing properties, but don't use more than an ounce a day of this powerful chlorophyll drink.

Some of my favorite juice combinations include carrot pear, kiwi pineapple tangerine, fresh ginger and apple, celery apple and lemon cucumber apple. You can create your own favorite combinations in the amounts that you are able to enjoy without having a reaction.

Carrot juice is popular but some people find that drinking too much of it brings the blood sugar up too high. If you have diabetes, hypoglycemia, or candida you should be especially careful about drinking too much carrot or fruit juice. Focus instead on juices made of mostly green vegetables and aloe vera, as well as vitamin C and garlic.

When beginning a juice program, start off gradually with perhaps an 8-ounce glass of juice three times a day, one half hour before meals. If you find your juice is too strong, you will need to follow it up with some water to dilute it. Do the same if you find your juice is too sweet and you feel fatigued after drinking it. You will then have to cut back on the sweeter fruits. After a week you can increase your juice and vegetable intake until you are consuming 30-40 grams of fiber a day.

The key to a healthy cleansing diet is to stay away from all animal proteins, saturated fats, sugars, processed foods, pesticides, fried foods, pickled foods and salted foods for a period of two months. After the first week you can rotate fish into your diet and increase the amount of grains and legumes. By starting the day with fresh juice and then a hot grain cereal you will be giving your body the essential nutrients it needs to rebuild and cleanse itself. Such a program will keep you satisfied and fit instead of leaving you hungry with cravings for unhealthy food.

The Gerson raw food and vegetable juice therapy. I give you this diet because a lot of people have benefited tremendously from it. Gerson primarily treated people with tuberculosis and then, later, cancer. The Gerson diet is without question the finest dietary approach to cancer that I know of. It has not helped or cured everyone but it has certainly had enough documented cases that it warrants respect. I believe that anything that can help people whose immune systems have been devastated with cancer regain energy would help with other conditions as well, and clearly that is the case with this program.

The program consists of about 13 glasses of fresh juices a day, primarily vegetable, for a period of about 2 months. The program is not excessively heavy on the carrot juice, because that can lead to a jaundiced condition of the skin. Rather, the juices emphasized are celery, cucumber, beet, lettuce, greens and apple. The juices and foods in this program are high in potassium and low in sodium. Also, fresh vegetable soups that are rich in potassium, and yogurt, whole grains, beans, seeds and starchy vegetables which help reestablish healthy bacteria in the intestines, are eaten.

Food supplements. While we need all the vitamins and minerals we can get from our food, I believe there are certain vitamins and minerals only available to us in supplemental form. On a cleansing program we should be taking on a daily basis 200-400 units of vitamin E, 2,000-10,000 mg of vitamin C, 200 mg of pignogenol, 2,000 mg of quercetin and 1,000 mg of NAC-inositolcysteine. In addition, we can take 200 mg of glutathione to help in the refortifying process. Be sure that your diet contains adequate essential fatty acids such as omega 3 and omega 6, which can be found in fish oil, flax seed oil, canola oil, walnut oil and oil of evening primrose. There are also beneficial antioxidants such as dioxyclor and homozone.

There are many other means of fostering detoxification for greater health. You may consider taking saunas (unless you have high blood pressure), or looking into homeopathy, acupuncture, mineral baths, reiki therapy, massage, chiropractic or aromatherapy. Intravenous vitamin C drips may help if you are seriously toxic or immune-suppressed. Also beneficial in relieving stress are meditation, yoga, guided visualization and the isolation tank. There are books available on each of these topics to help you familiarize yourself with these nontoxic ways of rebalancing your body chemistry.

The key to maintaining a good healthy body is to prevent the build-up of toxins in the body and resultant diseases. To meet this goal, the following substances, which can adversely affect health,should be avoided:

• Meat
• Dairy products
• Refined sugars
• Caffeine
• Tobacco
• Alcohol
• Recreational drugs
• Unnecessary medications
• Low- and high-level radiation
• Toxic heavy metals: lead, mercury, cadmium, aluminum, arsenic
• Toxic substances in the home/work environment
• Stress
• Parasites

CHAPTER 13

Clinical Experiences

The following section focuses on individual physicians as they discuss the specific tests and holistic treatments they use to help patients overcome health challenges. Their methods may be slightly different but their philosophies are similar in that they all believe the body plays an active role in restoring its own health. Dr. Charles Farr, in his assessment of bio-oxidative therapy, sums up the holistic approach to medicine when he says, "this treatment doesn't 'cure' anything, but helps patients to improve their level of health so that they can become less sick, since you cannot be sick and well at the same time."

Majid Ali, M.D.
Molecular Medicine: Intravenous Nutrient Protocols

Dr. Ali, of Denville, New Jersey, describes health as the molecular dynamics preserving the structural and functional integrity of cells, tissues and organs. Disease, on the other hand, can be defined as molecular events that result in cellular and tissue injury. Dr. Ali considers that the proper clinical practice of medicine is based upon these precepts of molecular medicine, and to this end he has developed a number of intravenous nutrient courses of treatment, or protocols, for a variety of conditions. None of the protocols consist of treatment with a single nutrient—all contain a variety of agents—and each is tailored to the individual patient and his or her unique condition. Also, the intravenous treatments are given in conjunction with other types of treatments appropriate to the patient.

Dr. Ali stresses that intravenous nutrient therapies make possible a dramatic reduction in the use of antibiotics and other types of drugs. He says that his protocols are "extremely effective for resolving hard-to-define but unrelenting clinical symptoms such as fatigue, a sense of being not healthy, stress and panic attacks, palpitations, mood and memory disorders, abdominal bloating, and symptoms of allergy and chronic sensitivity." He also finds intravenous treatments frequently effective in successfully managing patients with certain chronic degenerative and immune disorders who obtain little long-term relief from the drugs usually given for their conditions. And for some disorders for which there are no known effective drug regimes, such as incapacitating chronic fatigue, intravenous nutrient therapy can be quite valuable.

Dr. Ali emphasizes the difference between the study of the molecular dynamics in health and disease—or molecular medicine—and the study of the morphologic patterns of disease, which he terms "tissue injury medicine." "The issue of the use of non-drug protocols of molecular medicine versus the drug and surgical treatments is a critically important issue," he says. He draws the distinction thus: "The morphologic-diagnosis-established microscopic studies tell us about tissue injury after the tissue has been injured. The study of the dynamics of health and disease, by contrast, gives us insights into the workings of the cells and tissues before the injury has occurred. This indeed calls for a major intellectual adaptation. Like all other adaptations, it can be expected to create considerable difficulties for the physicians with intellectual subservience to classical medicine."

The Fallacy Of The Three D's

He goes on to explain that classical medicine follows what he calls the "dogma of the three D's"—one disease, one diagnosis, one drug. Drugs work by inactivating or impairing molecular pathways. This is what they are designed to do, and in acute, life-threatening disease, these molecular effects of drugs save lives, though often at a substantial cost in terms of adverse effects. In chronic immune-related and degenerative conditions, though, drugs carry a much higher potential for adverse effects, because they are used for longer periods of time, often for years. This is where nutrient protocols formulated with full knowledge of the structural and functional molecular relationships prevailing in health offer superior clinical benefits: The nutrients do not carry this risk of adverse effects.

Also, while drugs are essential for acute, life-threatening disease, Dr. Ali says that they are poor substitutes for nutrients when one wants to reverse chronic molecular disorders–depression, chronic fatigue and arthritis–referring to oxidative damage. He points out that while a hundred years ago, the major threats to the survival of our ancestors were imposed upon them by infectious agents, today, the major threats to our survival are imposed upon us by synthetic chemicals and toxic heavy metals, as well as by the stress of modern living. "The prevailing medical thought of the 19th century was dominated by the microbial threat," he says. "Today, the prevailing medical thought should be dominated by the oxidative threat. Regrettably, this is not the case at present. Why? Because we continue to seek answers to the medical problems of the late 20th century with early 19th century thinking."

Confronting The Front End Of Disease

Due to all the modern-day assaults on our cells, electron transfer defenses that ordinarily protect cellular health can fail. And, says Dr. Ali, "when these electron transfer defenses fail, the disease begins." Which tissue or organ turns out to be the seat of subcellular and cellular injury is determined in part by the patient's genetic make-up. Dr. Ali refers to the organ "elected by the body to break down" as the body's "spokes-organ." And he emphasizes that if we are seriously interested in preventative medicine, we must look at the front end of this process, i.e., molecular and energy events separating the state of health from the state of wellness.

Accelerated oxidative molecular injury is the "initial molecular lesion" at the beginning of all disease processes, Dr. Ali explains. He says too that "spontaneity of oxidation is the basic phenomenon which initiates the process of aging. The biochemical and cellular processes involved in aging can take place in a slow, sustained, and orderly fashion, preserving health for the length of the species life span. Or these processes can take place at an accelerated rate, causing disease and premature aging. This pacing, in my view, is a matter of central importance in our understanding of health and disease states. The compelling clinical concept here is this: All our therapeutic strategies for degenerative immune disorders, first and foremost, must be directed at reducing the need for increased oxidative molecular breakdown."

Dr. Ali explains that he uses intravenous nutrient protocols not to correct nutritional deficiencies, but rather to create a high gradient of nutrients inside and outside cells in order to meet the increased demands for these nutrients of tissues in various disease states. The intravenous route, bypassing the bowel mucosal barrier, eliminates all absorption problems. He uses intravenous treatment in conjunction with oral supplementation, and stresses that, in nutritional medicine, more so than in classical medicine, the metabolic individuality of the patient must be taken into account.

He uses nutritional therapy to treat a wide variety of conditions. These conditions include acute viral infections, where the commonly used antibiotics are of no significant value; acute, as well as chronic, disabling fatigue; asthma and incapacitating bronchospasm associated with pulmonary emphysema; autoimmune and immune-deficiency syndromes; and bacterial infections under treatment with appropriate antibiotics, the purpose here being to protect the tissues from drug toxicity.

What Dr. Ali refers to as "altered states of bowel ecology" constitute another condition that responds to IV nutrient therapy. These states include multiple food allergies, malabsorption problems, recurrent episodes of candida overgrowth, some types of colitis and parasitic infections. He also uses IV therapy for food and mold allergy that coexists with malabsorption, a circumstance generally associated with impaired absorption of oral nutrients; for heavy metal toxicity; and for musculo-skeletal pain syndromes.

Also, before and after major surgery, intravenous nutrient treatments are used to facilitate and expedite wound healing. The nutrients provide a counterbalance to the oxidative and other molecular stresses caused by the surgical procedures. Likewise, before and after chemotherapy and radiotherapy, intravenous nutrients are given to protect tissues from cell-damaging effects of the chemotherapy drugs or radiation.

Among the major nutrients used in the intravenous protocols are ascorbic acid, magnesium, cobalamin, pyridoxine and pantothenic acid. Dr. Ali calls ascorbic acid the "first-line-of-defense molecule" against oxidative stress to human tissue. Magnesium is another "miracle molecule" that can work as "nature's calcium channel blocker." Some other nutrients often used by Dr. Ali are vitamins A, D and E; biotin; folic acid; niacinamide; riboflavin; thiamine; zinc; and selenium.

The doctor also uses EDTA chelation therapy for reducing the body burden of toxic heavy metals and for reversing arterialsclerotic cardiovascular disease, integrating chelation with nutritional and lifestyle approaches to healing.

Health Hazards Of The Next Century

Dr. Ali sees a lot of patients with chronic fatigue and has written a book on the subject entitled, *The Canary and Chronic Fatigue*. He cautions that this condition cannot be understood through simplistic single-agent-single-disease models. One has to take a holistic view of the impact of the environment upon an individual's genetic make-up, he says, while looking at fitness-related factors, as well as nutritional status. He sees chronic fatigue as a state of accelerated oxidative molecular injury, and forecasts that this is going to be the dominant chronic health disorder of the 21st century. In fact, he predicts that it will be this disorder, more than any other, that will lead to the acceptance of intravenous nutrient therapy by the mainstream medical community.

Dr. Ali reports good-to-excellent results with IV nutrient therapy, citing, particularly, success in the treatment of acute viral pharyngeal and respiratory infections, asthma, fatigue syndromes and pain syndromes. In addition, patients facing surgery or recovering from it have benefited remarkably from IV nutrients, and he predicts that, as more physicians become enlightened as to the efficacy of this approach, it will become commonplace in hospitals.

Robert Cathcart, M.D.
Ascorbic Acid Against Free Radicals

Dr. Cathcart believes that the kinds of diseases most people suffer from these days come from multiple viral infections, chronic exposure to chemicals in the environment, and poor nutrition, all of which exhaust the free-radical scavenging system. He uses a comprehensive treatment protocol to eliminate pollutants and strengthen the system, with an emphasis on bowel-tolerance doses of ascorbic acid (ascorbate).

He explains that if there are ten people in a "sick" building but only one gets sick, there has to be a reason why that one gets sick while the other nine don't. So while it does help to clean up one's environment, the individual should also be alert to the possible need to clean up the multiple infections that may be exhausting his or her own free-radical scavenging system, such as candida and Epstein-Barr virus. In addition, there may be a need to reduce massive amounts of chemicals being taken in, and, generally, to improve poor nutrition.

Dr. Cathcart takes a multifaceted approach to eliminating negative elements from patients' diets and environments. He puts patients on an anti-candida program and takes them off sugars found in refined carbohydrates and processed foods. Then he tries to take them away from any known allergens. If they're living in moldy homes or working in sick buildings he attempts to take them away from those problem situations as well.

Strengthening Free-Radical Scavenging

Of course there are some viruses and chemicals that people just can't get away from. Dr. Cathcart tries to strengthen patients' own natural free-radical scavenging systems with vitamin C, vitamin E, beta carotene, zinc, manganese, chromium, and selenium. He also uses some amino acids, particularly cysteine.

The treatment he generally finds most helpful is administration of massive doses of ascorbic acid, to bowel tolerance. In fact, Dr. Cathcart stresses that when he refers to ascorbate, he is referring to the massive amounts of vitamin C that he gives for the electrons it carries. This approach goes far beyond the tiny amounts of vitamin C usually thought necessary for proper bodily functioning. "This is not the usual definition," he says, "and I only persist in this because I think there is a need to make this distinction. Since I'm the one who developed this titration to bowel tolerance, this gives me a certain right to define some things."

Dr. Cathcart has patients take the ascorbic acid orally, giving ascorbate intravenously only in acute situations or in situations where they can't handle it orally, as in the case of ulcer patients. He explains that since the effects of intravenous ascorbate last only a few hours, he always tries to work on increasing the amount of ascorbic acid patients can handle orally.

Treatment with massive doses of ascorbate has been highly effective, Dr. Cathcart reports. He says that when a patient who has been through the local doctor circuit comes to see him, if he makes that person well, it's probably 90 percent due to the ascorbate and 10 percent due to Dr. Cathcart's insistence about the patient's reducing sugar intake.

Bowel-tolerance doses of vitamin C absolutely relieve the acute self-limiting viral diseases, Dr. Cathcart says, referring to colds, the flu, mononucleosis and hepatitis. He finds hepatitis extremely easy to treat, noting that this is one of the situations in which he does use the intravenous route, because patients are usually quite sick when they come in with the disease, and results come a little faster that way.

Dr. Cathcart explains that to find out your bowel-tolerance dose of ascorbic acid, you should increase your dosage rapidly until you begin to get diarrhea. This isn't a painful diarrhea and it's extremely easy for people to do. Then take just a little less ascorbate than that amount. He says that for the typical person who is not sick with allergies but simply with a cold or the flu or some other infectious disease, there will be no difficulty whatsoever in titrating up to bowel tolerance and then feeling the effect of getting well from it.

Dr. Cathcart concludes that he never endorses anything other than ascorbic acid by mouth or sodium ascorbate by vein. "I find I cannot achieve these effects with the mineral ascorbate. The mineral ascorbates are very fine sources of vitamin C, so if a person had a disease due to a mineral deficiency the mineral ascorbates would be just fine. But we're not talking about vitamin C deficiencies here. We're taking about brutally neutralizing massive amounts of free radicals, and it's only the ascorbic acid that seems to carry enough electrons to be able to be taken by mouth to achieve this neutralization of these massive amounts of free radicals with acute illnesses."

Philip J. Hodas, M.D.
Cleansing The Brain

The brain becomes toxic due to its continuous exposure to some thousands of chemicals in our air, water, soil and food supply. We breathe 20,000 times a day, and if the environment is toxic and polluted, we breathe in toxins and pollutants.

Dr. Hodas explains that while nature has given us a blood-brain barrier to protect the brain from noxious substances, the constant inflow of chemical pollutants weakens and penetrates that barrier. Little toxins leak in, locking into brain cells and locking out nutrients. The result is a dual condition of both brain malnutrition and brain toxicity.

To say the brain is complex would be an understatement. The brain has its own anatomy, physiology, neurology, metabolism, bioelectricity, biomagneticity and biochemistry. It may weigh only 3 to 3.5 pounds, but it has 12 to 14 billion cells. (We utilize only 2 to 5 percent of our brain-cell capacity—7 percent for geniuses. A lot of our brain cells lie dormant, waiting for work.) We have four brain lobes: a front lobe, temporal lobe, parietal lobe and occipital lobe. Each lobe has numerous functions allowing us to live with some sense of organization, stability and balance, and to sense accomplishment and achievement. The left and right hemispheres are connected by a corpus callosum. Interestingly, the left hemisphere controls movements on the right side of the body; the right hemisphere controls movements on the left.

The brain, part of the central nervous system, also has a cerebral cortex, gray matter for thinking, a thalamus, and hypothalamus for feeling and emoting. Plus, it has a cerebellum for balancing, a pons, a midbrain, a medulla oblongata, and a spinal cord that comes out of the brain stem and attaches to a cord protected by vertebrae. *Gray's Anatomy* says the brain and central nervous system regulate all of our functions: balancing, coordinating, sensory input, receiving, storing, coordinating, integrating, remembering, retrieving, processing and utilizing information.

As to detoxifying the brain, there are a variety of approaches, says Dr. Hodas, some of which you can do yourself and some of which must be supervised by a physician. The physician should have a background in complementary, holistic, orthomolecular, nutritional, hygienic, metabolic, chiropractic or osteopathic medicine.

Taking Steps Yourself

Diet. Get a complete health and nutritional workup from a physician first. Then, you can go on to take dietary action yourself. Dr. Hodas recommends keeping a diary of what you eat for one week and writing down your symptoms. Over the next week, go on a transitional diet of steamed and raw foods and continue to note your symptoms in the journal. Drink only soups and raw juices, including watermelon juice. Have the watermelon apart from other food. Get lots of rest. Finally, reintroduce grains, legumes, fish, vegetables, fruits, nuts and seeds.

Once you start eating solid food it is important to go on a four- to five-day rotational diet to avoid overloading the immune system and developing allergic addictions, including brain allergies, to any foods. If you eat wheat on Sunday, for example, don't repeat it until Thursday.

Exercise. Do some aerobic exercises, such as jogging, jumping rope or using a trampoline, dancing, swimming, rowing or race walking. All will bring in some oxygen. Deep-breathing exercises also are helpful.

Vitamins, minerals, and amino acids. Antioxidants and other detoxifying nutrients are beginning to receive a lot of publicity in scientific circles and in the general community. The *New York Times* and other general-interest publications are beginning to carry articles on, for instance, the antioxidant vitamin E, and its benefit to people with heart disease. But this discovery is not brand new, Dr. Hodas notes. Health advocates such as the late Carlton Fredericks have been espousing vitamin E's advantages since the 1950s, and a number of books have been written on these benefits. Vitamin E, of course is just one of the many vitamins essential to our health. Others include: vitamin A, beta carotene, thiamine hydrochloride (vitamin B1), riboflavin (vitamin B2), niacinamide (vitamin B3), pantothenic acid (vitamin B5), pyridoxine (vitamin B6), folic acid (vitamin B9), choline and inositol (which make up lecithin), vitamin B12, vitamin B13, dimethyl glycine (vitamin B15), vitamin C, bioflavonoids, quercetin, rutin and pygnogenol.

Essential minerals include magnesium, zinc, manganese, sodium, potassium, selenium, glucose tolerance factor and chromium; and important amino acids include l-glutamine, l-cysteine and l-methionine. Essential enzymes include glutathione peroxidase, superoxide dismutase (SOD) and pancreatic and proteolytic enzymes papain and bromelin.

Other methods. Other methods Dr. Hodas mentions that may aid in the detoxification process, as well as help you relax, include taking mineral baths consisting of sodium, potassium and magnesium; learning transcendental meditation, or visualization; and using a flotation tank.

With Your Doctor

Concerning physician-aided ways you can detoxify, Dr. Hodas outlines several:

Chelation therapy. A physician can give you chelation therapy, which consists of EDTA (ethylene diamine tetra-acetic acid) administered via intravenous drip. You can also take nutrients for oral chelation, such as vitamin C, zinc and magnesium.

Amalgam removal. Have a holistically aware dentist remove your amalgam fillings and replace them with nontoxic ones. Amalgams release mercury into your system every time you chew.

Herbal cleansers and homeopathic remedies. Find a practitioner who understands how to use these therapies for brain and overall body detoxification.

Orthomolecular nutrition. "Orthomolecular" is a term coined by double Nobel Prize winner Dr. Linus Pauling. It means the right amounts of the right nutrients. You can go to a physician who practices orthomolecular medicine to get intravenous injections of nutrients in a drip, or intramuscular injections in a shot. Or you can take the supplements orally.

Other Treatments

A variety of therapies and substances can help detoxify the brain and rebuild it for better functioning, including biofeedback machines, massage, polarity, reiki, cell salts, herbs and Bach flower remedies. A doctor of acupuncture can help the detoxifying process by balancing your meridians to release blocked energies. Finally, the special field of developmental and behavioral optometry can help you reorganize the way you perceive space and think.

Christopher Calapai, M.D.
Getting To The Root Of The Problem

Dr. Calapai stresses the importance of getting to the basis of his patients' problems and not merely treating symptoms. He reports phenomenal success in many instances using a nutritional program fine-tuned to his patients' individual needs. And he emphasizes the importance of educating patients so that they can better understand what lifestyle changes are needed to keep healthy:

"I always begin by trying to understand what is going on with my patients," says Dr. Calapai. "Instead of waiting for patients to get sick and then trying to play catch-up medicine, or instead of waiting for them to exhibit symptoms and then treating only symptoms, I try to look for the causes of all the symptoms that the patient has." He goes on to point out that it doesn't make sense to just cover up symptoms, because then the problem will only manifest itself in other, more severe ways. And there may be several reasons for any one symptom. So it's important to look at all the causes of the problem, as well as to educate the patient as to what the body is or isn't doing.

Dr. Calapai puts a lot of emphasis on nutrition because he feels many people don't eat right. They may think they're doing the right thing by following a specific type of diet, and perhaps even adding some vegetable juices and vitamins, but their diets still may not be the right ones for them. For that reason, he always begins by having his patients undergo a series of tests.

Tests

Dr. Calapai does a blood test for all of his patients in order to get an idea of their vitamin and mineral levels, their digestion and absorption capabilities, and their cholesterol levels and fat intake. He has patients bring in a week's worth of their diet history so that he can see exactly what they're eating. Also, he tests people for food allergies to see of they're eating things over and over again that are causing them any number of delayed symptoms, or chronic ones.

"Fatigue is one thing I see most frequently with patients," says Dr. Calapai. "When we're looking for the cause of someone's fatigue we include a test for magnesium in the red blood cell. Studies in England have shown that low red blood cell magnesium levels significantly correlate with chronic fatigue, as do viral syndromes."

He relates the case of one patient who came in after having had all sorts of basic chemistry testing performed by another doctor. "We were able to find out the person had some food allergies as well as a low red blood cell magnesium. As soon as we took the allergens out of that person's diet and corrected the magnesium deficiency by using intramuscular magnesium shots, within about two weeks the person started to see significant improvement. The fatigue significantly decreased and was pretty much gone in about a month."

Allergies

After the preliminary tests and history-taking, Dr. Calapai puts the patient on a protocol free of junk foods, chemicals and preservatives, and devoid of food allergens.

He reports he's had good success with patients in overcoming allergy-related problems. "One such patient," Dr. Calapai says, "a gentleman in his early 40s, came to me with a history of aches and pains in the joints, and bowel problems. As soon as we started to use an allergy treatment on the individual, his joint pain went away. I was somewhat surprised, as was the patient. The patient couldn't believe that just by taking the allergy shots to the inhaled allergens he was able to see a dramatic change in what had been a chronic history of joint aches and pains. I suggested, just to test this, that he stop taking his allergy shots for the next couple of weeks to see what happens. He complied, and the aches and pains returned. We put him back on his protocol of once-a-week allergy desensitization shots, and the patient has been free of pain since."

Dramatic Improvements With Nutritional Changes

He's also seen a lot of dramatic health changes occur through simple changes in the diet alone. Such changes can optimize the cholesterol and blood-related picture: "Recently, for example, a gentleman came to see me with a ridiculously high cholesterol. I think it was over 300. After putting him on a diet without simple sugars but containing instead complex carbohydrates and good vegetable protein sources, the patient's cholesterol level dropped down to 150 or so."

Dr. Calapai says that when spectacular changes like this do happen, we really shouldn't be surprised. After all, it is what we put into our bodies that allows us to function—either well or less than optimally. "Simply by changing our diet around a little bit, instead of using medications to bring our systems under control, we can benefit immensely and feel truly well. I think that's the best way to go."

Jennifer Brett, N.D.
Naturopathy

Dr. Brett is a naturopathic physician practicing in Stratford, Connecticut. She explains that naturopathic medicine is somewhat of an umbrella term meaning that naturopathic physicians help the body heal itself through a variety of natural methods. Depending on the practitioner, that might include herbal medicine, nutrition, hydrotherapy, homeopathy, colonics or any combination of treatments. She explains her approach to diagnosing and treating patients:

"The assessment I use is similar to that used in conventional medicine in terms of taking a complete history and giving a physical exam. I then try to find the cause of the illness, disease or discomfort. A chronic headache, for example, might be due to an ongoing exposure to a chemical at work, or it may be due to a sluggish metabolism causing digestion to take place very slowly." In any case, she always asks herself, "What is it that causes this person to have discomfort?" in order to help the person through treating the cause rather than the symptoms.

Arthritis

When anyone comes in with a chronic illness of any sort, Dr. Brett says, the first thing she does is help the body with elimination. "I use mostly herbal medicine for this. I've seen people with rheumatoid arthritis, for example, where I've started out by using cleansing herbs to detoxify the colon and the liver. The inflammation decreases dramatically.

"Then I try to find what substances are causing the increase in inflammation. One client of mine works on car bodies," she adds. "The paint fumes and the metal chips and probably other substances were causing him inflammation. The long-term treatment in his case, because he wasn't willing to give up his work, was to develop an air filtration system in his workplace so that he wouldn't constantly be bombarded by these products. As a result the arthritis in his neck and shoulders has decreased tremendously."

AIDS

Dr. Brett feels that naturopathic practitioners are getting more and more comfortable working alongside conventional practitioners with debilitating diseases, such as AIDS or cancer. She feels there can be good interaction between the two groups, because naturopathic physicians offer treatments to help the body's immune system heal while more conventional therapies work to attack the illness.

In fact, Dr. Brett points out, a recent issue of the *Journal of Naturopathic Medicine* was all about treatments for HIV-related infections of various sorts. Usually AIDS patients are given dietary modifications to improve their health through vitamin, mineral and herbal supplements. Then they are given a range of choices with which to work in terms of long-term help. These choices may include hydrotherapy, fever therapy, counseling, support groups or other choices. "Each individual has something that will work for him that may or may not work for the person next door," says Dr. Brett. "So what we try to do in the naturopathic community is find something that will feel good emotionally and physically. Physically, can you swallow 25 vitamin pills a day? If not, then that's not the way we should go in this case. What can we do in terms of food that will help you? And so on." The idea is that when treatments are individualized, the protocol works better for each individual than if it was cookbook-type medicine.

Steven Bock, M.D.
Holism For Multiple Symptoms

Dr. Bock, of Rhinebeck, New York, has been practicing holistic medicine with his brother Ken for 15 years. He notes that in the past few years he has been seeing patients with increasingly severe problems from toxic exposure to such things as pesticides, bad water and other pollutants, as well as poor nutrition and high stress levels. People's systems, especially their livers, he explains, are overloaded and having a harder and harder time getting rid of toxins.

The typical patient he sees exhibits multiple symptoms: There usually isn't one clear-cut problem to treat. Instead, most patients have many minor symptoms they learn to live with. Dr. Bock points out that traditional medical training doesn't teach doctors how to work with such patients. So he has investigated on his own and learned ways to help bring people's bodies back to a state of health—first through getting rid of what he calls "the bad stuff" (toxins) and then by helping them function at the best level they possibly can with the aid of good water, good food, good air and spiritual energy. Finally, he tries to help the body maintain its homeostasis.

Dr. Bock describes the typical patient who comes to him:

"The cases I see generally focus around immune problems— allergies, chronic fatigue, intestinal problems—or things like headaches, PMS and other chronic symptomatology. When you go into people's histories you usually find that in addition to their having headaches they might have gas, bloating, allergy symptoms, weight problems and energy problems. They need to sleep a lot, or they feel exhausted at a certain point of the day. I compare these people to a rain barrel too full. They have lost their reserve capacity. They're overflowing with toxins down the front, back and sides of the pail, depending upon the day's stress levels, allergens, environmental exposures, etc. Their systems are reacting but in a general way."

Dr. Bock stresses that the body has a certain homeostasis in health and also a homeostasis of maladjustment. "It resets its thermostat so it's in the best balance given the situation." People he sees in a chronic state of poor health usually have many symptoms across many systems. For instance, they have energy problems and mental problems, perhaps confusion and memory problems. Often their gastrointestinal system may be affected with diarrhea and bloating. They may have difficult urination or cystitis. In addition, they may have such conditions as nasal stuffiness, post-nasal drip, chronic sore throats, swollen glands, wheezing and shortness of breath. "In other words, they have symptoms that don't fit into one diagnosable category such as asthma."

The First Step: Detoxification

"I usually begin helping people by having them go on some kind of detoxification program," says Dr. Bock. "I might want them to begin with a fast. Sometimes I have people use a product like UltraClear, which is a metabolic clearing diet that works extremely well in helping people reduce their toxic load. I'll do that for a two- or three-week period. At first, they'll be on a modified fast, where they won't eat food for three days, and then they'll eat very hypoallergenic, simple foods that won't tax their systems.

"If I'm looking at someone whose problem is limited to their GI tract, I might have them go on a GI detox using a bentonite preparation. Bentonite is a very fine clay substance that absorbs toxins. I'll have them follow that with psyllium husk, which gives a mucilaginous cleanse to the GI tract. A GI detox is important because if the GI tract isn't functioning, the whole system isn't getting nutrition. That will complicate any illness by not allowing the person to replenish nutrients."

Another part of the body Dr. Bock pays close attention to is the liver, because it plays an important role in eliminating poisons and performs many other vital functions, such as manufacturing proteins, distributing blood sugar, and breaking down hormones.

To test symptoms that might be related to liver function, such as PMS or headaches, he brings in some of his acupuncture training. Acupuncture looks at the body differently than Western medicine does, the doctor explains, in that it looks at certain meridians. There's a gallbladder meridian, a liver meridian, a kidney meridian, and so forth, and Dr. Bock will examine patients from that perspective. "Symptoms and a physical acupuncture exam let you know that a person has certain excesses or deficiencies in certain organs. For instance, a patient comes to me with symptoms of headaches on the sides of the head, PMS, digestive problems and flank pain. They may also have tinnitus and a bursitis of the hip, gas and pain in the right upper quadrant. All those symptoms are related to the gallbladder meridian.

"The liver meridian, located on the inside of the leg, regulates a lot of symptoms women often have, especially pelvic problems. So if someone exhibits such symptoms along with tender liver meridian points, I might come to the conclusion that the person's liver meridian is really overloaded. Then I might use a liver detox, such as some Chinese herbal remedies. Other herbs I use to cleanse the liver include dandelion and milk thistle."

Another area in need of detoxification, says Dr. Bock, is the lymph drainage system. When a person is reacting to a lot of things, lymph problems can usually be detected. These problems can result from antibiotics. Dr. Bock treats a lot of Lyme disease patients, and in these cases a person must take antibiotics. "When you treat a Lyme disease patient, you'll sometimes find that they get better with some of their main symptoms, such as their neurological symptoms, palpitations and headaches. But they'll have a flare-up of a lot of general symptoms. This occurs because when you destroy spirochetes, you're breaking them up into little pieces. All of a sudden, instead of handling one bad germ, your body has to handle ten. It doesn't know if the shells of the spirochetes are not alive and therefore reacts to them the same as to living germs. You may have overloaded the circuit and you need to detox from that."

The system clears by having the lymph pick up waste, Dr. Bock explains, sending it through the lymph glands and out through the bloodstream. To help the lymph drainage system, he often uses homeopathic remedies, and finds they're generally helpful.

He notes that you can also release toxins effectively by sweating them out in sauna treatments. This is recommended in helping people get rid of pesticides and volatile petrochemicals.

"I doubt that we will ever be able to overcome environmental pollution by fighting the powers that be because we are run by the industrial corporations," says Dr. Bock. "So I think on an individual basis we have to work to eliminate allergens, to help the lymph drainage and liver, and do other important things to help ourselves."

Dr. Bock relates the case of a typical patient. "A 38-year-old woman came in to see me who said that she had been feeling fatigued for the past eight years. She went to internist after internist but to no avail. Finally, one doctor told her that she might have chronic fatigue, but he didn't explain what that was. He told her there was no treatment for it other than to rest.

"She came to me and I found out that she was eating poorly and was a stressed-out, type-A person. She was showing signs of weakness related to blood sugar problems and chronic fatigue, among other things. In addition, her system was chronically toxic and had about ten things wrong with it. She had vertical disease rather than horizontal disease. In other words, she was walking around sick instead of being hospitalized.

"I told her that she needed to change her diet in order to get the proper vitamins. But first she needed to clear her system and I explained the general cleansing program using UltraClear powder followed by a rotation diet.

"Her first reaction was to resist the change. The first thing she said to me was, 'If I do that, does that mean I have to eat that way for the rest of my life?' I had to help her set milestones by seeing things in the short term. I said, 'Why are you thinking about what you need to do for the rest of your life when we haven't even gotten you better yet? Let's concentrate on getting you better in one month.'

"A month went by and her health was much improved. Over the

course of three months she was a totally different person. Now I don't see her much anymore, except for an occasional follow-up visit, because she's gotten to a much better level of health." Dr. Bock adds that the patient has come to understand that, yes, one does have to make healthier dietary and lifestyle changes for the long term; going on a temporary "diet" just won't do the trick. But once you see a change in your health, the notion of compliance becomes a different concept, one that is much easier to live with.

Conditions

Food addictions. Approximately 60 percent of the people who come to see Dr. Bock have some form of allergy; very commonly those addictions are to foods. Allergy usually indicates that your system is unbalanced and that your body is operating in a mal-adaptation mode. He explains that sometimes a better word to use is "sensitive," because this process is not reflected by the standard allergic mechanisms like IgG and IgE. Your body gets affected by sugar, caffeine or wheat, for example, and if you eat those foods you get a certain kind of symptom. You might get racy and hyper. Or you might feel fatigued. You have an addiction and withdrawal pattern.

The addiction stimulates certain receptors on particular body organs and actually increases receptor sites. The cells always crave the filling of those receptors. So in order to stop the addiction you need to be able to give the receptors certain things to fill that craving. You may have to do exercise, for example, or to undergo behavior modification counseling to learn what to do. You might be advised, for example, to go running before you eat.

An addiction to sugar usually means that the carbohydrate metabolism—usually involving the liver and adrenals—is really having problems. Dr. Bock usually gives sugar-addicted patients nutrients to help support the liver. Also certain minerals are given, like magnesium, zinc and potassium for the adrenals. He gives vitamin C too, for detoxification, and pantothenic acid. "I prime their system by helping them to detoxify, and I support them nutritionally." Basically, he is orthomolecularly trying to push the body away from the maladaptive state of addiction.

Dr. Bock will often add acupuncture to a patient's treatment because acupuncture is good at balancing the body, especially when someone has anxiety, sleeplessness, palpitations or nervousness. "They can be anxious, and when you give them a treatment, ten minutes later they're asleep. It elevates their endorphins and it fills those receptors so that they don't have cravings and they don't have any of the problems they were having."

Hypertension. He treats hypertension by looking at each person's individual profile. If the person is a type A who has really driven himself, he uses a lot of relaxation therapy. Then there are a whole variety of protocols to choose from, depending upon the patient. "We use chelation therapy in our office. And nutritionally we treat patients with a lot of antioxidants like vitamin C, garlic, vitamin B-6 and vitamin E. The exception is in certain cases of hypertension where you have to watch out for vitamin E because it elevates the pressure. Part of our practice involves tailoring nutritional needs to individual cases of hypertension and cardiac problems."

Holistic Medicine Is Empowering

Dr. Bock says that since he's started helping people detox and improve their level of health through diet, homeopathy, acupuncture and other natural means, patients have been coming to understand how they themselves affect their health. "If you say to people they have a particular disease, people feel disempowered. But if you communicate to them by saying, 'This is your system and your system is doing the best that it can given where you're at; we're just going to get it to a better state of functioning,' people feel more connected to the process."

Helping People Who Are Ready To Change

"We still have people come into our office who aren't ready to try holistic medicine. Most of our practice is holistic, but we're one of the few offices that integrates conventional and holistic medicine in a family practice. In one sense we want to educate people. On the other hand, we're not going to shove things down people's throats. So if someone comes to us and they're not ready to look at acupuncture and they're in pain, we use analgesics."

Dr. Bock reports that a lot of M.D.'s don't know about holistic medicine but that some are gradually opening up to it. "Both my brother and I are board-certified physicians and still have a hospital practice. We interact with a lot of our colleagues and while they may perceive us as strange, they know we perform well in the hospital and in our offices. Some of them are referring difficult cases to us.

"I had a patient the other day who was referred to me by her gynecologist because of severe pain with intercourse. He had given her a battery of tests and she was even laparoscoped. Finally, he said to her, 'I did everything I can do,' and sent her to me. I told her and her husband about acupuncture and they didn't really believe me but she decided to try it anyway. I did treatments on her liver and the problem disappeared. When the couple came back, the husband, a very pragmatic, skeptical sort of person, admitted that her problem was gone and his whole opinion about acupuncture had changed.

"It's really interesting when you see someone who is 75 years old open up to holistic medicine. I saw a woman who was operated on by an orthopedist. Afterwards she was in chronic pain. She had bursitis on the side of the leg and back pain. Her doctor tried her on Motrin and Naprosyn but nothing worked. Luckily her conventional doctor, a friend of mine, said, 'Look, I've done everything. I can't think of anything else. Why don't you see Dr. Bock?'

"She came in for acupuncture not knowing if it would work. After the treatment, she got off the table saying, 'I don't believe this.' She was walking around while her cane was hanging on the hook of the door. Her husband was saying, 'Margaret, you're not using your cane!' You could see the look in their eyes as they started to believe in this concept for the very first time. It's very gratifying to see people change this way."

I-Tsu Chao, M.D.
Tackling Food Allergies

Dr. Chao, whose practice is in Brooklyn, New York, has been doing independent research on allergens and treating patients successfully since 1959. According to the doctor, most, if not all, chronic conditions stem from food allergies. These include chronic urticaria (hives), arthritis, respiratory problems, headaches, chronic fatigue and even backache and menstrual problems. He helps patients determine the substances to which they are allergic and to activate their enzyme systems so that they no longer have problems metabolizing those foods. Dr. Chao explains his methods of testing and treating patients:

Provocative Testing

"First we find the cause of the problem. One method we use is called provocative skin testing. We challenge the patients with antigens and find out what they react to. Usually people have problems metabolizing food. Incompletely metabolized foods become antigens or foreign bodies and the immune system reacts to them, causing inflammation and diseases due to allergies."

Activating Enzyme Systems

Dr. Chao will then reverse the allergies with what is called neutralization treatment. For example, if a person is allergic to milk, you dilute milk into a 1:25 dilution or a 1:125 dilution and you give this to the patient. This activates the enzyme system, says Dr. Chao, and all the patient's symptoms disappear within ten minutes. The doctor goes on to explain that while people do call this process neutralization, it is not actually neutralizing; it is, rather, activating the enzyme systems to metabolize the foods completely.

"Once we activate the specific enzyme system, all the food is metabolized and there are no more foreign bodies. Consequently, the body requires no more immune response. If there is no immune response there is no inflammation. No inflammation means no more disease."

People with asthma, for example, says Dr. Chao, usually have a chronic cough, wheezing, a stuffy nose and post-nasal drip. When they have something they are allergic to—milk, for example—their symptoms soon follow. "If we do a skin test we can reproduce these symptoms. And if I find a good right dosage of this same milk to activate the related enzymes, the patient can function normally. All the milk will be metabolized and all the symptoms will disappear. No more stuffy nose, no more runny nose, no more coughing and the wheezing stops. The patient will be able to drink milk without trouble.

The same kind of testing and treatment apply to other foods— e.g., wheat, corn or rice—and to other substances, such as dust, pollen or mold in the air. Once body functions are restored to normal the body can break down all the foreign bodies and metabolize substances completely. Then it becomes possible to eat food without trouble and even inhale the pollen in the air without trouble. Medication is no longer necessary, says Dr. Chao, and you can lead a normal life. You can exercise, you can garden, you can do anything you want. Weather changes will never make you sick. You won't catch colds any more because your body has built up resistance. All your body systems will function normally.

"Before these treatments every allergic food produces foreign bodies—incompletely metabolized food metabolites—within the body. So your immune systems have to work harder to take care of these foreign bodies (unwanted substances). That's why if you are suffering from food allergies you always have low resistance since your immune forces have to fight off multiple enemies. You can catch colds and get infections easily. Once I normalize the body function, the immune system is ready to fight off any virus or bacteria. You have a very strong resistance to the infection."

Preserving The Enzyme System Through Food Rotation

Dr. Chao usually tells patients not to eat the same thing every day, but to rotate foods. This helps preserve the body's enzyme system because if you eat the same food repeatedly the same enzyme is used over and over and you exhaust that body function. Then, when the food is eaten again, the body cannot metabolize the food and it can get you sick. "My idea," says Dr. Chao, "is that every food is good if you don't eat it every day. Every food is not good if eaten all the time."

Along with diet, he usually recommends that patients take high doses of vitamins C, E and A, and minerals. He reports that through a combination of activating the enzyme system and rotating and supplementing the diet, he usually helps 99 percent of his patients.

Specific Conditions Related To Food Allergy

Candida. Cravings for sugar usually signify a yeast problem, says Dr. Chao, and it probably means infection with candida. If you take care of the candida the cravings for sugar will also disappear.

"Usually I can do this by getting the immune system to control the yeast population. I use a candida extract to activate the body's enzyme system; the body's immune system also becomes active and takes care of the yeast overgrowth. For acute yeast infections, I usually have good results in a few days using the candida extract more frequently."

Hidden allergies. Many times patients don't realize that certain problems are related to food allergy," says Dr. Chao. "Low back pain, for example, is almost always related to food allergy. Most of my patients have backaches but come to see me for something else. I tell them from the beginning that their backache will disappear along with the asthma or whatever. And it does. The same time the asthma or whatever disappears so does the backache—even if they've had it for 10 or 20 years.

"The same thing is true for female problems. Painful menstruation, dysmenorrhea, is related to food allergy. When I take care of the food problems the menstrual pain disappears as well. Morning sickness is also related to foods. When I help a woman for something else, she has no more morning sickness. Also, women going through menopause should never feel sick. When a woman has trouble, it's always from food. She's not supposed to have any symptoms. She should be comfortable. If she has any type of trouble it's from food, usually from common foods that she eats every day.

"At first I had no idea that these things were related to allergy but I've observed this over the past 30 years. People who were helped—people with other conditions—would tell me that they were no longer having trouble with their menstrual periods or backache. So this was actually discovered accidentally. I didn't expect it in the beginning."

Arthritis. Dr. Chao says that whenever anyone suffers from arthritis, regardless of the form it takes, food is always involved. Usually the person has trouble with every food. He concedes that this is not a popular point of view. "But after 30 years," he says, "I've found this to be the rule, not the exception. I can help these people through the same method: I help activate their enzyme systems to that they can eat food without trouble."

Emotional and mental health. "Allergies affect the nervous system and brain and thus our mental and emotional states. Some of these conditions manifest as nervousness, anxiety, epilepsy, hysteria and mania, schizophrenia and other forms of mental disease. Criminal behavior is related to diet too. So is hyperactivity. If we get the foods right, our body will function normally. And not only will we have a healthy body, but a healthy mental and emotional condition as well."

Dr. Chao believes that when people become really good at making radical, lasting changes, it may be possible for them to live to

160 or 170. "But first, people's concepts have to change. If we can help people to change their eating habits, we can create a happier, healthier society."

Wyrth Post Baker, M.D.
Homeopathy

Dr. Baker, of Chevy Chase, Maryland, trained simultaneously in allopathic and homeopathic medicine at Hahnemann University to get an understanding of both theories of medicine so that he would be able to treat patients more effectively. He uses homeopathic remedies 90 percent of the time.

Testing Patients

"We start off by doing a complete diagnostic study, giving a physical examination and taking a complete history of our patients. Then we do supplementary laboratory studies, the usual hematology, blood chemistry, thyroid and any specialized studies that we deem essential to pinpoint any particular disorder."

Treating Symptoms, Not Diseases

Dr. Baker prescribes, for the most part, according to homeopathic methodology by selecting one or several homeopathic drugs that seem to be most applicable to the particular symptom picture being treated. "Part of that has to be done by intuition and experience beyond the book," he explains.

"We do not treat disease. We treat on the basis of symptomology. Different diseases may have similar symptoms. The same disease may have a wide variety of symptoms. So the selection of the best indicated homeopathic medicines depends on how closely we analyze the particular symptom picture. We then select medicines from the pharmacopoeia and the materia medica that have the most similar picture."

Dr. Baker explains that homeopathic drugs were originally tested by giving them to essentially normal individuals who were studied to see what symptoms they produced. A careful record of those symptoms was made, to be used as a guide as to how to use the drug.

"By giving the best indicated drug to a patient, we attempt to re-establish homeostasis. When the body is in perfect homeostasis it's essentially well. When some part of the physiology gets out of this homeostasis then some disorders appear. It may be called a disease, it may be called any number of diagnostic terms.

"We try to find the particular drug that produces the basic symptomology that the patient presents, studying, of course, the objective findings as well as the subjective symptoms that the patient has. The more carefully we select, naturally, the better the results will be."

Advantages Of Homeopathy

At Hahnemann University Dr. Baker trained in both allopathic and homeopathic medicine, and he feels it was the broadest education he could get. Since then he has been using homeopathy on about 90 percent of his patients. "The main advantage of homeopathy is that you are dealing with substances that are not toxic and that never produce poisonous effects. And if you don't help the patient at least you don't do anything to hurt them. You don't have drug reactions when you use homeopathy. It doesn't always cure every condition, naturally, nor do any of the drugs. But when it is given and prescribed carefully, the results are quite favorable. It does not replace allopathic medicine entirely, but we have to learn where it is indicated, where it's likely to succeed, and with which cases it's likely to fail. When we know the properties and the ill effects of our drugs then we can select intelligently to get the best results without unfavorable results. It's a matter of knowledge and experience."

Nicholas Gonzalez, M.D.
Battling Serious Disease Through Life Changes

Dr. Gonzalez, of New York City, is a medical doctor specializing in immunology. He sees mainly cancer patients—about 70 percent—but also treats people with other disorders such as multiple sclerosis, lupus, chronic fatigue, Epstein-Barr virus and arthritis. He uses an aggressive nutritional protocol combining various detoxification protocols, nutrition and supplementation.

"We offer a very unorthodox approach emphasizing nutrition. As opposed to using orthodox treatments such as chemotherapy or radiation, we work strictly with a holistic approach that involves three different areas: diet, nutritional supplementation and detoxification. Each person's program is individualized, but generally speaking, the diet consists of organic and unprocessed foods, and the nutritional supplementation involves taking between 100 and 150 capsules per day of different vitamins, minerals, amino acids, glandular extracts and enzymes. Specific foods and supplements depend upon the results of the patient's laboratory tests."

Dr. Gonzalez uses a detoxification protocol that involves getting rid of any waste material, including tumor breakdown products that have formed, with the idea that if you don't get rid of them they can keep you toxic. Practically speaking, that means that the patient does daily coffee enemas. Other detoxification protocols take place within the treatment, but each one is individualized. Some of the other protocols involve a liver flush, a "clean sweep" protocol, a purge and rubbing of the skin from head to foot with mixtures of olive and castor oils that Dr. Gonzalez believes the body uses to excrete waste material through the skin, salt and soda baths, mustard and food soaks and castor oil compresses.

Patients come to see Dr. Gonzalez in all stages of disease. As a rule, he says, the earlier a person comes in after the original diagnosis, the more that person can be helped. But there's not one particular stage in which the doctor accepts or doesn't accept patients. "We take each case individually. We do a prolonged interview with each patient to evaluate the case—to determine whether or not we can benefit the patient—taking into consideration such things as the time of original diagnosis, the extent of metastasis, the kind of organ involvement, the kind of previous treatments the person has had, if any surgery was performed, if the patient is taking any kind of medications or drugs, if they're able to eat, able to get around, pain level, if the person smokes, things to that effect."

A Rigorous Program

For lasting success, Dr. Gonzalez believes people must completely change their lives. He stresses that his program is a life-changing one, and most patients change the way they eat. It involves taking supplements up to six or seven times a day, including waking up in the middle of the night to take pancreatic enzyme. It means doing coffee enemas two to three times a day at times. It's a very aggressive, rigorous program. But he says that chemotherapy is not any easier.

We find that success is directly proportional to their level of compliance. But again, we will try not to accept a patient into our program unless we really feel that they can benefit from it. We don't want them coming in, paying all the money, and going through all the different details of the program if we don't think we can help."

Ronald Hoffman, M.D.
AIDS And HIV Treatment

Dr. Hoffman has a holistic medical practice in New York City. Here he discusses successful treatment protocols for helping patients with AIDS, HIV and other immune-related diseases: "The protocol we use really varies according to a person's immune status. We're more aggressive with patients who seem to be in a decline phase with HIV. Initially people are in a latent phase where they just remain with the virus present in their systems. Then they go through a period of relatively rapid decline. When we see patients begin the decline phase we initiate more radical therapy.

"Initially the therapy can be as simple as dietary modification and oral vitamins. Patients can remain on the therapy for months or years and remain in a good holding pattern. The highlights of that therapy are the antioxidant and immune-augmenting nutrients such as vitamins C, A and E, selenium and zinc. These are the crucial basic foundation nutrients we use. We also use more esoteric things such as licorice extract, which we now import from Japan under the name of glycyrrhizin, extract of shiitake mushroom, and the bioflavonoid quercetin, which has a potent anti-HIV effect. We incorporate these nutrients to keep people's immune systems stable. We often add garlic as well, because garlic is an important nutrient for enhancing the natural killer cells. These are oral nutrients that we might use.

"The nutrients I just mentioned are members of the antioxidant family. Interestingly, they have a dual effect. They prevent free-radical damage to cells and they enhance the immune system; they seem to regenerate systems that help the body fight infection. One of the things we see in HIV patients is a decline in the effectiveness of antioxidant systems. We often find a reduction in the level of glutathione, which is present in the lungs and tissues and defends against infection. By providing the antioxidant nutrients, particularly selenium, we can enhance that defense system. There is also a new antioxidant we like to use with HIV patients, N-acetyl-cysteine. It's being tested on a scientific basis as a means of preventing some of the consequences of HIV infection. It's very effective in enhancing the antioxidant defense and it may have a direct antiviral activity against the retrovirus that causes AIDS."

Dr. Hoffman generally suggests that people refrain from using preservatives of any kind. He thinks that even in normal people with normal immune systems these things are devastating. In people with an immune problem, they have an especially devastating effect. So his cardinal rule is no junk, no preservatives and an avoidance of sugar (except in some people who are suffering from a wasting syndrome where he might give them protein supplements with natural sugar to boost their calories). He doesn't espouse a vegetarian diet because he no longer believes, as he once did, that a macrobiotic diet is the be-all and end-all of HIV treatment. He says that while many patients can benefit from a macrobiotic diet if they do it skillfully, many are miserable on it and perform the diet poorly. He therefore recommends a diet that includes fish and poultry, taking care, when people have lower T cell counts, to give them special precautions about avoiding foods that might carry parasites, fungus or bacteria.

Pannathpur Jayalakshmi, M.D
Helping The Chronically Ill

Dr. Jayalakshmi received her basic medical degree in India in 1962 helping the chronically ill. She did her post-graduate work at Hahnemann University. She practiced traditional medicine for 17 years before becoming very ill and helping herself with natural therapies. She currently has a holistic medical center in Philadelphia that incorporates colonic and chelation therapy and other nontoxic approaches to cleansing and rebuilding health.

Thorough Detoxification

"The type of patients we see here are usually the people who have gone everywhere else and not found results," says Dr. Jayalakshmi. "Most of the time they come here as a last resort. Very few patients—about 10 percent—are prophylactic and pediatrics. Mostly they're here with chronic degenerative diseases: cancer, hypertension, diabetes, arthritis, allergies, asthma, chronic fatigue syndrome and AIDS.

She emphasizes nontoxic therapies and focuses on lifestyle: nutrition and very thorough detoxification are stressed.

"We help the detoxification organs of the body—skin, liver, thyroid, kidney and colon. Many times we recommend a person start out with a detoxifying diet. Such a diet differs depending upon the patient's situation. Sometimes we recommend a juice fast and a cleansing diet of raw foods. And sometimes a maple/lemonade fast or honey and lemon water fast.

"To help the colon we encourage people to take colonics. The colon is a very large organ; it's a six-foot-long tube. The residues that accumulate there become very toxic to the body. Normally we should eliminate three times a day but very few people do that. So the colonics help. We also suggest eating high-fiber foods to help increase bulk, such as bran."

Another organ of detoxification is the kidney, Dr. Jayalakshmi says. To help here, she encourages patients to drink a lot of fluids. And for the skin, she suggests skin brushing, sweating and exercise. "For the lungs we encourage proper breathing through breathing exercises. We also detoxify the liver and thyroid. For the whole body we recommend stretching exercises, sometimes even yoga." More than anything, though, she says that the mind is extremely important, so she recommends stress-reduction techniques.

Chelation Therapy

"Chelation is available for everybody unless a person has a severely damaged liver or kidney or brain or something like that. Otherwise, everybody is a candidate. People can use chelation even as a prophylaxis. It removes the heavy metals from the body. All of us have a higher level of heavy metals in our body compared to primitive people. Since it removes the heavy metal, it creates cellular homeostasis. It makes every cell function better."

She notes that chelation is particularly helpful for vascular problems: intermittent claudication, heart diseases, stroke and angina. "We see many angina patients. After five, six or seven chelation treatments their chest pain disappears and they need less drugs. They practically take no drugs. Many people with high blood pressure are given drugs to take for the rest of their life. After receiving chelation and changing their lifestyle, their pressure comes down to normal and they need no more drugs. These are people whose blood pressures were not controlled in spite of several drugs. Now—with no drugs—their pressures remain normal."

Success Stories

"We have innumerable cases of people who have improved through our methods," says Dr. Jayalakshmi. "You can use me as an example. I used to be so sick before with migraines. I was working in the city of Philadelphia and I had to park the car on the road and get out to vomit many times or lie down in the car to rest. I was so sick that I felt my life was not even worth living. That is the state in which I was once upon a time. Now, 14 years have passed and I feel so great that I'd like to go on and on as long as God wishes me to.

"We help cancer patients improve their health. We had one patient here with a breast tumor. By the time she came she had already had a mastectomy done on one side. She also had a tumor on the other side. She did not want to go through surgery. She was on this program and within two weeks she noticed that the tumor had regressed. She went to her gynecologist, who was surprised that the tumor had disappeared. She simply said, 'Do whatever you're doing; it's fine.' Then this lady had many stresses in her life and didn't continue the program. She slacked off and became over-confident. The next time she went for a checkup the tumor had reappeared. She was startled and became frightened enough to carefully resume her program. She went back for her next checkup to find that the tumor was no longer there. So she was almost playing with the appearance and disappearance of her malignant tumor depending on the way she was following the program. Now she follows the program carefully and is surviving and thriving.

"We see many patients with AIDS or who are HIV-positive. They are all under control. We have even seen situations where patients reverse back to normal. Their T-4 count improves and reverses to normal."

Dr. Jayalakshmi sees many chronic fatigue patients as well, including many people who have very good positions in life but are on disability because they cannot function. "When those people come to us they gradually get better and better and better until they can resume working again." With her chronic fatigue patients, in addition to helping them cleanse and rebuild their systems in the usual way, Dr. Jayalakshmi uses one additional product: intravenous dioxychlor, a nontoxic synthetic substance to kill the virus.

"Success is directly proportional to how good people are in following their lifestyle changes," Dr. Jayalakshmi stresses. "If a person changes their lifestyle and sticks to the program, which includes stress reduction, then the success rate is 100 percent."

Dorothy Calbrese, M.D.
Countering Chemical Sensitivities

Dr. Calbrese, of San Clemente, California, graduated from Columbia College of Physicians, Surgeons in New York City, where she studied pediatrics. She changed her field of specialization, however, to allergy/immunology due to her own need to overcome a major health challenge caused by severe chemical sensitivities.

"I grew up in New York, where I became sensitive to many chemicals in the city's environment. I lived near a plant in the Bronx which exposed me to a lot of pollution. I also seemed to be very sensitive to chlorine and a lot of the chemicals they added to the regular water supply. In addition, I was sensitive to chemicals added to foods. After graduating from medical school, my husband and I decided to start a family. I found that with each pregnancy I got sicker and sicker. I started going to various hospitals and seeing lots and lots of specialists. . . . It turned out that I was highly allergic and chemically sensitive.

"Most of the patients I see tend to have a genetic predisposition toward being chemically sensitive. In this practice, a lot of patients have thyroid disease. There seems to be some basic problem associated with prostaglandins, fatty acid metabolism and thyroid function that tends to either aggravate or get the chemical sensitivity rolling. We rarely see people who are very chemically sensitive who don't have laboratory, radiographic or sonographic evidence of clear-cut thyroid disease, even though it may be secondary."

Allowing Nature To Heal

Dr. Calbrese's treatment involves using nutrition and helping people to cleanse by doing such things as eating organic food, breathing clean air and drinking good water. That works very well, she reports. "A lot of detoxification programs consist of taking vitamins and all sorts of things. But many of the patients I treat are just way too sensitive to vitamins and to lots of detoxification methods to do that. So what we're doing is focusing on rebuilding the immune system in terms of immunotherapy, and then just cleaning out and letting nature heal itself. For our patients who are severely incapacitated, we send them to Dr. Rea, who has a program set up involving saunas and other methods to help with major detoxification."

The kinds of recommendations she makes to patients to maintain health are lifelong. Drinking a lot of pure water is essential. Some people can drink distilled water, she says, although that's not the best method for most. "Some people can drink good water from a pure source, bottled in glass. Some people can even handle regular filtered water if the filter is a very good one. It depends on how sensitive the individual is. In a normal person, who doesn't have cardiac or renal restrictions or some other disease that restricts fluid intake, we recommend at least eight glasses of water a day, but most of them are drinking more.

"In terms of air, we have a real problem. In southern California—I'm right between Los Angeles and San Diego, which used to have some of the cleanest air in the country—the air quality has something to do with weather pattern inversions. Even the coastal area outside of the metropolitan area is very much affected by the air pollution. We recommend that people try to get to places where they're further apart from their neighbors so that they don't have the immediate pollution from their neighbors' chimneys and other things. We also recommend they live higher up. I live 2500 feet up on a mountain, where the air is tremendously clean. But many people in southern California have to work here and don't have the luxury of just picking up and leaving. For them air filters can be helpful but they don't really do everything. There's no question that the cleaner the environment in which your house is located, the better."

She often recommends changes within the home environment. She likes patients to get away from things like carpets, drapes, wood-burning stoves, gas and using pesticides and other chemicals in the home, pointing out that many products are not necessary once you learn to replace them with nontoxic products. "We go very much more toward a long-term clean-living kind of approach."

She sees varying degrees of improvement in patients, with many doing very well. "You have to remember that by the time people get here they've usually been on medicines. They've usually seen lots of doctors and they're usually doing very poorly. That's why they're still looking for another approach. Because of that they're extremely motivated. The other thing is that we only take people who we think are going to do well. Of course our results are excellent because we're screening people to see who we think are going to do well and who are very motivated. I think the key to the whole thing is that patients really need to understand themselves very well and they need to find the doctor who is best suited for them.

And then the doctor needs to be very selective about the patients they take. I think in this economy doctors often are not, and that causes problems. If you take the people who are best suited for this kind of thing then you get very good results.

"The kinds of results you see: People, many of whom were totally disabled from arthritis, asthma, chronic fatigue or any of a whole host of illnesses, return to work. They may even start a whole new career, get married and just get on with a normal life. They get on, they're happy and things go well for them. It is easy for them to be compliant long-term when they see cause and effect."

Dr. Calbrese cautions that if you expose yourself to the things that made you sick, you will definitely go back down. "There's no question that someone like myself—and I'm as bad as most patients I'll see—is never entirely right because the genetics never change. There was a lot of construction today on the road when I was coming to work and I was exposed to a lot of diesel exhaust. It didn't make me sick as it used to because I'm in clean air most of the time. But most people wouldn't have even noticed the smell.

"You have to follow the lifestyle that's going to help you long term. It's a question of just using good common sense. You don't get a heart attack, go through cardiac rehabilitation and then just go back to being a couch potato and not paying any attention to your diet. You really need to stay on top of it. When you're sick it's hard to do these things, but when you make these changes and you feel so good it's easy to stay on top of it."

Emotional Support

Emotional support is often lacking among the patients' family and friends, Dr. Calbrese warns. "It's enough to make you think you're crazy when you have these kinds of problems as it is. There's a tendency to say that many of the patients' problems are psychiatric when in fact these are just regular people who have a genetic predisposition toward certain diseases or who have had a toxic exposure to something and have become ill. It's very depressing—no matter how confident you are or how successful you've been—when you have these kinds of problems and people don't understand them and don't know what to do for them. It's difficult and people need support."

For this reason she sends a lot of patients to the Viscott Center. The center, begun by psychiatrist David Viscott, author of *Emotionally Free,* uses a simple, straightforward approach that has been very helpful in supporting patients emotionally. She notes that he's good at helping patients get back on track, with one or two visits. Also, she tries to screen out psychiatric patients so that they get appropriate help.

Lifestyle Changes: The Best Insurance

"There's no one answer for everyone," Dr. Calbrese points out, "no one way to find help. People have to live a lifestyle they like, and people have to live in a way that keeps them happy and healthy. That takes a huge amount of work and it's expensive to begin with. Eventually it becomes less expensive but in the beginning it's very expensive to make all these changes. People may have to move and do all sorts of things. If they do it and it's extremely successful, and in most cases it is, it will reinforce the changes."

Dr. Calbrese feels that making appropriate lifestyle changes is the only answer to the health care debt we're going to be creating over the next decade. She says that medical care will get more restrictive for older patients as certain diseases become excluded from coverage because they're not as easy to treat. But she says, "People who have done major things to optimize their health at ages 20, 30, 40 and 50 will not be burdened with, 'Gee, if I have a heart attack maybe I'll be over the age limit for getting treated,' as is the case in other countries such as England where they don't treat certain people with these problems as they get older because it's not cost-effective." She concludes that optimizing one's own health early is the only thing for an intelligent person to do at this point.

Dr. Louis Parrish
The Parasitic Plague

Dr. Louis Parrish of New York has done extensive research on parasites for the past 20 years and concludes that the problem is more widespread than people realize: Parasitic infections are not just a problem for third world countries with tropical climates; they infect people everywhere. Approximately one out of five New Yorkers suffers from parasitic infections, and is unaware of it.

What Are The Symptoms Of A Parasitic Infection?

Dr. Parrish discusses the problem in detail: "Protozoa are little one-celled animals—amoebas and giardias—that we get in our gastrointestinal tract when we eat contaminated food or drink polluted water. Recently in New York, for example, there was a problem with the *E. coli* bacteria in the water. When there is a problem with *E. coli*, following that there are going to be these little one-celled animals."

Dr. Parrish explains that the pathology caused is a local erosion or destruction of the mucosa of the gastrointestinal tract. There are so many symptoms associated with infection by *Giardia lamblia* and *Entamoeba histolytica* that he links the two together, referring to them as the protozoal syndrome because a patient usually has them both.

"Outside of the local pathology in the gut, besides increasing or decreasing its motility or eroding the mucosa so that there is malabsorption of essential nutrients, there are other symptoms." Infestation can affect the immune system because the giardia do their damage in a part of the duodenum that manufactures over 50 percent of the secretory immunoglobulin. That cuts down the number of antibodies produced. "But there are so many things associated with this syndrome that you're unable to explain it by any pathogenesis that might arise from the destruction or interference with the normal functioning of the GI tract: bloating, gas—and the gas is, particularly with *giardia*, frequently foul—erratic bowel movements, or sometimes the system goes to extremes, from constipation to persistent diarrhea.

"People think of amoebas as actually physically invading the liver. They don't invade, but interestingly they sometimes cause a type of nonspecific hepatitis. And this is recognized among establishment doctors. This has to be due to a toxin. In the old literature, yes, they will say that there is a toxin release, but they attribute this to secondary bacterial infiltration of the erosions or ulcers made by the protozoa. That's in the literature. But it doesn't explain patients coming in, for example, with obvious disturbances in the blood sugar level. One simple example is sweet cravings. I would say 8 percent, to be fair, present with a chief complaint of sweet cravings. Now if you treat something specifically with a medicine that only affects one type of microbe and the symptom goes away, you can begin to deduce they're related. So the sweet cravings go away. But they also have a very peculiar life cycle and they're not telling anybody what governs it, whether it's the moon or the stars or the weather or what. Then if it comes back after treatment and they start the sweet cravings again, you treat them with the same specific medicine, and you have proved your deduction by replication."

Dr. Parrish notes that the protozoal syndrome can cause emotional and cognitive symptoms, including memory loss. "You really can't think clearly. The motivation is down. One of the reasons, of course, can be psychological because you don't have the energy to do what you want to do to participate in life. You don't even have the time or the good humor. You lose friends because you're irritable. Is that because you're sick. I think it's because of a toxin."

Dr. Parrish explains that, because many patients describe their general condition with this infestation as being a feeling of toxicity or of being drugged or in never-never land, not caring and not having the strength or physical and mental energy to get up and get started again, he ascribes this syndrome to a chemical toxin.

He goes on to mention *cryptosporidium*, a small protozoan causing a disease called cryptosporidosis. This disease is one of the major opportunistic infections attacking AIDS patients, further depleting their energy when it's already decreased.

He explains that parasites have two stages of life. "In biology class, do you remember seeing something moving under the microscope, sending out little limbs and retracting them? That's a type of amoeba. They extend their arms and grab a red blood cell, bring it back in, grab some dead bacteria, bring it back in. As their energy fades they grow tired. They can't sustain themselves, and outside they can only live for an hour. So they surround themselves with a hard crust to form a cyst which many people think of as an egg. Right before they encyst, they burrow into the superficial mucosa of the bowel, make themselves a little burrowed tunneled-out ulcer which is typically flask-like. That is, they go into the hole and set down under the lining. There they build a hard shell around themselves and procreate. Then they get out, sometimes get into the bowel and attach outside with this crust.

"They can live for up to two weeks in freezing temperature. And this was always called a tropical disease until recently! No, it's not. First of all, if you had that little trophozoite as soon as it hits the stomach acid it's done with. With the crust of the cyst it can pass right through until it hits the alkaline duodenum, until it bursts open and we've got a new trophozoite around each nucleus. Then they start their dirty work.

"The *giardia* live in the upper part of the small intestine in the duodenum where most of the essential nutrient functions go on— absorption of all the trace elements and vitamins and so forth. In that 10 to 12 inches they can do a lot of damage. That's why it's important to have supplements.

"Then the amoeba, Entamoeba histolytica, makes its home in the ulcer in the large bowel. Besides releasing a toxin, I think they erode the flat plates of the sympathetic and parasympathetic nervous systems, which is why you get constipation. Or if they're agitated you get diarrhea."

Dr. Parrish says that parasites can affect every aspect of your life. Besides causing gastrointestinal problems and fatigue, the irritation of the cysts can precipitate the symptoms of cystitis prostatitis and PMS, and cause low-back pain.

How Widespread Is The Problem?

Dr. Parrish estimates that in Manhattan, for instance, at least one out of five people is infected. "A lot of these people travel abroad. But that's not where the problem is. New York is almost as epidemic as Morocco because of our food handlers. Any immigrant here— not matter what his background or education—the first job he usually gets is working in an eatery of some sort. And many can't read the advice to wash their hands. Furthermore, most come from cultures where it's just not the custom to wash your hands after using the bathroom, and I'm not talking about urinating.

"I did a little study one time. I was at a health fair. It was at the Sheraton on Seventh Avenue, which is a good hotel. These were people half from the Expo and the other half from a car company or something like that. I paid the attendant and said to him, 'What I want you to do is to count the number of men who go into the stalls and count the number who flush the toilet before they exit, and then see how many wash their hands.' Fewer than half who were deduced to have had a bowel movement went and washed their hands. You have to take away another 10 percent of men who didn't want to stand next to each other at the urinal and things like that. Of course there are variables in estimating the numbers, but regardless, the figures were impressive enough."

Beaver Fever

Dr. Parrish discusses a condition commonly called beaver fever, which started over 10 years ago in the Adirondacks in upstate New York. "People were getting *giardia*. They traced it back to beavers going to the bathroom in those crystal springs in the Adirondack Mountains. I've talked to several rangers from there who said they spend more time trying to keep people from drinking the water than they do showing off the beautiful scenery. And where does the water go from the Adirondacks? Down the Hudson, into the Catskills, Poconos, Delaware Water Gap and into the reservoirs. The Catskill Reservoir is one." He adds that patients from Canada are now coming to see him. "I'm finding out that the lakes north of Toronto or Ontario are loaded with beaver fever."

How Do You Stop The Problem?

Dr. Parrish gives patients literature to acquaint them with all the facts, but says that parasites are a hard subject to deal with because you're talking about what many feel are alien creatures. "Furthermore, if I call a patient and he wants to give me a progress report, the first thing he'll say is 'let me close the door.' He doesn't want anybody to hear about it."

He goes on to caution that there is no miraculous cure. "It's a treatable, controllable condition, but I'm not going to use the word 'cure.' That's because in most of the people I see, the infestation has gone on for so long that the bugs have burrowed in and settled down. So you've got to root them out. And instead of making medicines, they're taking them off the market. That's why I made an herbal product.

"Everybody knows about *E. coli*. I've cited references in the *New York Times*, *Newsday* and everyplace else. But nobody wants to touch it because so much money is involved in fixing the water supply. I don't think people like to talk about the subject. You wouldn't want me to say you had a guest over, he used your bathroom and didn't wash his hands, and contaminated your clam dip, would you?"

Additional Clinical Experiences

Some alternative doctors who, for a variety of reasons, are reluctant to be quoted in a book, nevertheless employ therapies and espouse beliefs readers should be informed of. Some of these follow.

Testing

One doctor always performs a hair analysis to measure mineral levels in the body and see if there is heavy metal poisoning, as well as a blood test. He also performs tests with a machine from

Germany called the Bio-Electro Meter of Professor Vincent (BEV) that gives him an idea of the state of the patient's immune system by analyzing the blood, urine and saliva. This doctor reports that the BEV machine was designed some time ago by a professor in France who studied the effects of water and found that where the water was worst there was the highest incidence of cancer and degenerative disease. Conversely, the best water sources were correlated with the lowest incidence. The BEV is used to assess nine nutritional parameters that can affect the immune system. Results are put through a computer to produce a nutritional outline.

Another test sometimes used is contact reflex analysis. This is something chiropractors do; the idea is that through testing muscle reflexes in the body one can find out everything that's wrong with the body, and whether the problem is emotional, structural, nutritional or biochemical. Then a determination can be made as to how to correct the problem.

Chronic Fatigue

An extremely common condition doctors see is chronic fatigue syndrome. One doctor, who says that this is in fact the problem he sees most frequently, reports that he uses injections of vitamins B6, B-12 and folic acid; liver; adrenal cortical extract, which is a natural extract containing all the hormones in the adrenal glands; and AMP, which turns into the energy molecule ATP in the body. He injects that twice a week intramuscularly.

A regular protocol he uses for chronic fatigue is to test for the Epstein-Barr virus. For patients with Epstein-Barr or a lot of fatigue he may use garlic or lysine, or hydrogen peroxide to release oxygen. To help the immune system and the intestinal tract, he also uses things like shiitake and reishi mushroom and a powder made from whey, along with acidophilus. Germanium, co-enzyme-Q10, carnitine, vitamin B-15 and zinc are also helpful, he adds, in destroying the Epstein-Barr virus, strengthening the immune system and raising energy levels. Potassium and magnesium aspartate can be valuable as well.

Allergies

Allergies can be tested for and treated in a number of different ways. Sublingual testing with drops is sometimes used. Another approach is testing a patient's pulse to make a neutralizing dose for allergies based upon what the patient needs. There is also a technique involving adjusting acupuncture points and reprogramming the brain so that the person no longer reacts to the allergens. A spring-loaded gun is used to adjust certain points in the spine, resulting in an eradication of the allergic response.

High Blood Pressure

One of the main causes of high blood pressure, according to a doctor who treats this condition, is metals in the liver, such as lead, cadmium, copper or chromium. These accumulate in the liver and stress it, affecting the blood vessels. Chelation therapy is used for this problem, as are garlic, herbal diuretics and lifestyle changes, which can involve diet, exercise, giving up caffeine and learning better ways to deal with stress.

Cancer

If a person's immune system is compromised from cancer, one doctor says, the most important thing is to cleanse the liver, blood and colon, as one would do for any other degenerative disease. To help the liver, this doctor does a liver gallbladder cleanse with apple juice or water, olive oil and lemon juice. The person drinks this for three days. He adds a certain amount of phosphoric acid to help soften the sludge and get rid of any stones in the gallbladder or liver. The doctor explains that this is not really a fast, but rather a regimen to flush out the gallbladder and liver while eating lightly, which causes the gallbladder to contract and to release toxins.

For colon cleansing, a series of colonic hydrotherapy irrigations can be used in conjunction with a nutritional program consisting of vitamins, minerals, enzymes and herbs. Changes in the diet and lifestyle are made at the same time if it is determined from tests that the person needs this.

To cleanse the blood the doctor sometimes uses homeopathic remedies and things like garlic and chlorophyll. Intravenous hydrogen peroxide treatments, which are sometimes used for patients with chronic fatigue, Epstein-Barr, yeast and emphysema, may be used for those with cancer as well.

HIV And AIDS

A doctor who treats HIV and AIDS patients says that the kind of treatment given depends on whether the patient is in the initial, latent phase of HIV, or in a decline phase. Initially, treatment can simply be dietary modification and oral vitamins. Antioxidant and immune-building nutrients, such as vitamins A, C and E, selenium and zinc, are given. Other substances given are glycyrrhizin (licorice extract); extract of shiitake mushroom; garlic; quercetin, a bioflavonoid that has an anti-HIV effect; and the new antioxidant N-acetyl-cysteine. This doctor stresses that patients can remain in the latent phase of HIV for months or years using these nutritional therapies.

When patients start to go into a decline, this doctor begins intravenous vitamin C therapy, and he reports that it often will help stabilize T-cell counts.

Some doctors use ozone therapy for HIV. This bio-oxidative treatment—accepted in Europe but controversial here—seems to enhance the immune system and inhibit viral replication.

Careful attention to diet is stressed by a holistic doctor treating AIDS patients. Dietary vigilance means that nothing injurious to the immune system should be eaten—no preservatives, no junk food and no sugar (except for some patients with wasting syndrome, who benefit from natural sugar as a calorie-booster). Another dietary concern: Patients with low T-cell counts who include fish and poultry in their diets should take special precautions to avoid foods containing parasites, fungi or bacteria.

Doctors using natural therapies for HIV patients have reported long, asymptomatic "holding patterns," dramatic increases in T cell counts and even changes of HIV status from positive to negative.

Other Therapies

A treatment used by some doctors for arthritis, musculoskeletal disease, multiple sclerosis and gout is bee venom therapy. Purified venom is injected, simulating a bee sting. This stimulates the immune system and adrenal glands to stimulate cortisone, and is said to improve circulation and oxygenation of the body.

One doctor uses a treatment called neurotherapy, which involves injecting procaine or lidocaine. He reports that neurotherapy is a natural treatment that helps restore the nervous system, and uses it to alleviate low back pain and other problems due to trauma by restoring the normal electrical charge on the nerves. He also finds neurotherapy of value in treating all kinds of headaches, including migraines, and for sinus problems.

Electromagnetic considerations are stressed by some doctors, who advocate a sleeping position in which the head is facing north and the feet south, in line with the electromagnetic charge of the earth. Patients are advised to modify their bedroom surroundings so that electromagnetic radiation doesn't adversely affect their health. They are told, for example, not to sleep on a water bed or too close to a digital clock.

CHAPTER 14

Overview

When we look at the world in which we live, we can no longer accept that there are single chemicals, foods or pollutants, each causing single diseases. Rather, we have to take the more comprehensive point of view, realizing that we live in a sea of contaminants—probably more than 100,000 all told—and that our bodies are filled with viruses and bacteria, parasites, yeast and fungi. Some of these are positive, but many are destructive, and whether we ultimately manifest disease or wellness will depend in large part upon the attention we pay to the status of our health vis-à-vis these various microbes and pollutants.

So we have to make a choice. If we choose to become indifferent, deciding that we are helpless to do anything about our health, and that we are simply going to be hopeful that we don't get sick, we have, in essence, chosen to play Russian roulette. If, on the other hand, we choose to make a constructive effort to see what we can do to minimize our exposure to those toxins over which we have control—e.g., by drinking bottled or distilled water instead of tap water; by eliminating sugars, animal proteins, most dairy products and processed and pesticide-laden foods from our diets and replacing them with organic and more natural and wholesome foods; and by using healthier and more ecologically correct building materials instead of asbestos- and formaldehyde-contaminated ones—then we've chosen to be far healthier than those who assume that what goes into their body doesn't matter.

There is no longer any puzzlement about what causes disease. We know what causes disease. We know, to a large extent, what prevents disease. And so we know, if we want to prevent disease, or at least to elevate ourselves from the Russian-roulette mode of daily existence, what we can do for ourselves. We can do a nutritional assessment to determine the levels of heavy metals in our systems and see whether these could be interfering with our enzyme systems and causing everything from mood swings to liver dysfunction.

We can take those vitamins, minerals and herbs that will stimulate a healthy immune response by cleansing and detoxifying the body's tissues of pollutants. And, of course, we can change our diets, eliminating red meat and chicken, lessening or eliminating dairy products, reducing our fat intake to 15 to 20 percent of total calories, eliminating sugars, caffeine, cola beverages, fried foods and excess calories, and putting an emphasis on fresh, organically grown produce. We can increase our fiber intake to at least 30 grams/day and eat at least six servings of fresh fruits and vegetables daily, including lots of juices. Finally, we can combine all these positive steps with regular aerobic and anaerobic exercise to strengthen the muscles and the cardiovascular system, and we can learn appropriate ways to deal with stress.

This program may sound like a lot to do. It is. One does have to exert oneself to be healthy. But looked at in another way, fostering our health is just a matter of making the right choices. Yes, we do have to break some old habits, and go through some temporary discomfort. But then we gain a whole new sense of wellness. Besides, fostering our health is the only way to go for those of use who plan to be around in the year 2020—and not just be around, but be around in great shape!

The bottom-line question is this: Isn't it time, in our fight against disease, that we stopped looking for single-cause excuses to blame, or silver bullets for cure? Neither have worked for us. What works, rather, is a comprehensive examination of life and our role in it, coupled with a seeking of the place that we can choose to begin our own healing process. What's involved is awareness, education, reading, questioning and—most important—active participation.

In fact, all of the doctors and others who have guided people who were at death's door—turning them in the other direction and helping them regain life through education, discipline and focused action—have emphasized that active participation by the patients was what made the incredible turnarounds possible.

Participation is the key. It's what environmentalists and nutritionists have been stressing for decades. And it's only now that average Americans are catching up and realizing that it is in their interests to do the same.

Endnotes

Introduction (p. viii-ix)

1. "30 Years Since Silent Spring," *NYCAP News* (New York Coalition for Alternatives to Pesticides), Early Spring 1993, p.7.

2. Charlene Laino, "With Cancer Rates Up, Environment Is Blamed," *Medical Tribune,* April 29, 1993, p. 8.

3. Ibid.

Chapter 1 (p. 8-13)

1. "Safe Ozone Levels Said to Increase Asthma Risk," *Medical World News,* May 1992, p. 9.

2. Earl Lane, "Ozone Thinnest Ever in '92," *New York Newsday*, April 23, 1993.

3. Eugene Linden, "Who Lost the Ozone?", *Time*, May 10, 1993, p. 56-8.

4. Dan Fagin, "Sick Buildings Face Senate Cure," *New York Newsday*, April 23, 1993, p. 47-8.

5. Ibid.

6. The Associated Press, "Solvent Used at IBM Tied to Miscarriages," *Daily News*, June 9, 1993.

7. Lawrence K. Altman, M.D., "Outbreak of Disease in Milwaukee Undercuts Confidence in Water," *New York Times*, April 20, 1993, p. C3.

8. Ibid.

9. Matthew L. Wald, "High Levels of Lead Found in Water Serving 30 Million," *New York Times*, May 11, 1993.

10. Associated Press, as cited by *New York Times*.

11. "Vital Signs," *World Watch*, May/June 1993, p. 6.

12. Keith Schneider, "Administration to Freeze Growth of Hazardous Waste Incinerators," *New York Times*, May 18, 1993, p. A1.

13. Keith Schneider, "For Crusader Against Waste Incinerator, a Bittersweet Victory," *New York Times*, May 19, 1993.

14. Schneider, "Administration to Freeze Growth of Hazardous Waste Incinerators."

Chapter 2

1. Balfour, C.B., **The Living Soil,** Devin-Adair, New York, 1952.

2. Borgstrom, George, "Food and Ecology," *Ecosphere*, The Magazine of the International Ecology University, 2 (No. 1): p. 6, 1971.

3. *Environmental Science and Technology*, 4 (No. 12): p. 1098, 1970.

4. Gerras, Charles, and others (editors), **Organic Gardening**. Bantam Books, New York, 1972.

5. *The Statistical Abstract of the United States*. Grosset & Dunlap, 1975.

6. Thomas Jr., William L. (editor), *Man's Role in Changing the Face of the Earth*, University of Chicago Press, 1956.

7. **Man in the Living Environment,** The Institute of Ecology Report on Global Ecological Problems, 1971.

8. Journal of the American Water Works Association, June, 1950.

Chapter 3

1. "30 Years Since Silent Spring," *NYCAP News*, (New York Coalition for Alternatives to Pesticides), Early Spring 1993, p. 7.

2. T.T. Iyaniwura, "Non-target and Environmental Hazards of Pesticides," *Rev. Environ. Health*, 1991 9(3), p. 161-76.

3. *NYCAP News*, p. 7.

4. Dan Fagin, "Cancer Causer: Study Shows DDT Residues Increase Risk," *New York Newsday*, April 21, 1993. p. 7.

5. "Pesticide Use: Agriculture Is King," *NYCAP News*, Late Summer 1992, p. 10.

6. Keith Schneider, "DuPont Plans Inquiry on Pesticide Crop Damage," *New York Times*, June 17, 1993, p. A23.

7. D. Godon et al., "Incidence of Cancers of the Brain, the Lymphatic Tissues, and of Leukemia and the Use of Pesticides Among Quebec's Rural Farm Population," *Geogr. Med.*, 1989, 19, p. 213032.

8. D. Godon, P. LaJoie and J.P. Thouez, "Mortality Due to Cancers of the Brain and Lymphatic Tissues and Leukemia as a Function of Agriculture Pesticide Use in Quebec, 1976-1985," *Can. J. Public Health*, May/June 1991, 82(3), p. 174-80.

9. P. Vineis et al., "Exposure to Agricultural Chemicals and Oncogenic Risk," Med. Lav., September/October 1990, 81(5), p. 363-72.

10. K.M. Semchuk, E.J. Love and R.G. Lee, "Parkinson's Disease and Exposure to Agricultural Work and Pesticide Chemicals," *Neurology*, July 1992, 42(7), p. 1328-35.

11. L.M. Brown et al., "Pesticide Exposures and Other Agricultural Risk Factors for Leukemia Among Men in Iowa and Minnesota," *Cancer Res.*, October 15, 1990, 50(20), p. 6585-91.

12. J.E. Davies, "Neurotoxic Concerns of Human Pesticide Exposures," *Am. J. Ind. Med.*, 1990, 18(3), p. 327-31.

13. B. Weiss, "Behavior as an Early Indicator of Pesticide Toxicity," *Toxicol. Ind. Health*, September 1988, 4(3), p. 351-60.

14. D.S. Rupa, P.P. Reddy and O.S. Reddi, "Clastogenic Effect of Pesticides in Peripheral Lymphocytes of Cotton-Field Workers," *Mutat. Res.*, November 1991, 261(3), p. 177-80.

15. R.M. Whyatt, "Setting Human-Health-Based Groundwater Protection Standards When Toxicological Data Are Inadequate," *Am. J. Ind. Med.*, 1990, 18(4), p. 505-10.

16. C.K. Winter, "Pesticide Tolerances and their Relevance as Safety Standards," *Regul. Toxicol. Pharmacol.*, April 1992, 15 (2 PT 1), p. 137-50.

17. "Cancer From Our Food: Ms. Browner Meets Mr. Delaney," *NYCAP News*, Early Spring 1993, p. 6.

18. Ibid.

19. "U.S. Pesticide Labeling Audit Reveals Many Problems," *NYCAP News*, Early Spring 1993, p. 17.

20. Fagin, *New York Newsday*, p. 7, 103.

21. "PCBs, DDT and Breast Cancer," *NYCAP News*, Late Summer 1992, p. 7.

22. M. Teufel, I. Vohn and K.H. Niessen, "Exposure of Our Children to Pesticides, PCB and Potentially Critical Anions," *Monatsschr. Kinderheilkd.*, August 1991, 139(8), p. 442-9.

23. "Ozone Depletion Caused by the Pesticide Methyl Bromide," *NYCAP News*, Late Summer 1992, p. 26.

24. S.H. Zahm and A. Blair, "Pesticides and Non-Hodgkin's Lymphoma," *Cancer Res.*, October 1, 1992, 52 (19 Suppl), p. 5485s-5488s).

Chapter 4

1. R.D. Benz and H. Irausquin, "Priority-Based Assessment of Food Additive Data Base of the U.S. Food and Drug Administration Center for Food Safety and Applied Nutrition," *Environ. Health Perspect.*, December 1991, 96, p. 85-9.

2. S. Green, "Research Activities in Toxicology and Toxicological Requirements of the FDA for Food and Color Additives," *Biomed. Environ. Sci.*, December 1988, 1(4), p. 424-30.

3. H. Babich and E. Borenfreund, "Cytotoxic Effects of Food Additives and Pharmaceuticals on Cells in Culture as Determined with the Neutral Red Assay," *J. Pharm. Sci.*, July 1990, 79(7), p. 592-4.

4. A.K. Giri et al., "In Vivo Cytogenetic Studies on Mice Exposed to Orange G, a food Colourant," *Toxicol. Lett.*, December 1988, 44(3), p. 253-61.

5. A. Maekawa, et al., "Lack of Carcinogenicity of Tartrazine (FDC) Yellow No. 5 in the F344 Rat," *Food Chem. Toxicol.*, December 1987, 25(12), p. 891-6.

6. A. Roychoudhury and A.K. Giri, "Effects of Certain Food Dyes on Chromosomes of Alliumcepa," *Mutat. Res.*, July 1989, 223(3), p. 313-9.

7. E. Novembre, "Unusual Reactions to Food Additives," *Pediatr. Med. Chir.*, January/February 1992, 14(1), p. 39-42.

8. K.M. MacKenzie, et al., "Toxicity Studies of Caramel Colour III and 2-acetyl-4 (5)-tetrahydroxybutylimidazole in F344 Rats," *Food Cem. Toxicol.*, May 1992, 30(5), 417-25.

9. G.F. Houben et al., "Effects of the Colour Additive Carmel Colour III on the Immune System: A Study with Human Volunteers," *Food Chem. Toxicol.*, September 1992, 30(9), p. 749-57.

10. M. Hannuksela and T. Haahtela, "Hypersensitivity Reactions to Food Additives," *Allergy*, November 1987, 42-8, p. 561-75.

11. M.A. Lewis et al., "Recurrent Erythema Multiforme: A Possible Role of Food Stuffs," *Br. Dent. J.*, May 20, 1989, 166(10), p. 371-3.

12. G.A. Settipane, "The Restaurant Syndromes," *N. Engl. Reg. Allergy Proc.*, January/February 1987, 8(1), p. 39-46.

13. D.A. Moneret-Vautrin, "Monododium Glutamate-Induced Asthma: Study of the Potential Risk of 30 Asthmatics and Review of the Literature," *Allerg. Immunol.* (Paris), January 1987, 19(1), p. 29-35.

14. C. Furihata et al., "Various Sodium Salts, Potassium Salts, A Calcium and An Ammonium Salt Induced Ornithione Decarboxylase and Stimulated DNA Synthesis in Rat Stomach Mucosa," *Jpn. J. Cancer Res.*, May 1989, 80(5), p. 424-9.

15. M.C. Wu et al, "Perserved Foods and Nasopharyngeal Carcinoma: A Case Control Study in Guangxi, China," *Cancer Res.*, April 1, 1988, 48(7), p. 1954-9.

16. L. Tollefson, "Monitoring Adverse Reactions to Food Additives in the U.S. Food and Drug Administration," *Regul. Toxicol. Pharmacol.*, December 1988, 8(4), p. 438-46.

17. B. Wuthrich and T. Huwyler, "Asthma Due to Disulfites," *Schweiz. Med. Wochenschr.*, September 2, 1989, 119(35), p. 1177-84.

18. W.C. Howlend III and R.A. Simon, "Sulfite-Treated Lettuce Challenges in Sulfite-Sensitive Subjects with Asthma," *J. Allergy Clin. Immunol.*, June 1989, 83(6), p. 1079-82.

19. S.L. Taylor et al., "Sensitivity to Sulfited Foods Among Sulfite-Sensitive Subjects with Asthma," *J. Allergy Clin. Immunol.*, June 1988, 81(6), p. 1159-67.

Chapter 6

1. Martin, W.C., "When Is Food a Food and When a Poison?," *Michigan Organic News*, March, 1957.

2. J.A. Goldman, et al., "Behavioral Effects of Sucrose on Preschool Children," *Journal-Abnormal-Child Psychology*, December 1986, No. 14(4), pages 565-577.

3. Ibid.

4. Strong, L.A.G., **The Story of Sugar**, George Weldenfeld and Nicolson, London, 1954.

5. Ibid.

6. Dufty, William, **Sugar Blues**, Chilton Book Co., Radnor, Pennsylvania, 1975.

7. Lyons, Richard D., "Sugar in Almost Everything You Eat," *New York Times*, News of the Week in Review, March 11, 1973.

8. Himsworth, H.P., *Clinical Science*, 1935.

9. Banting, F.G., *Strength and Health*, May-June, 1972.

10. Consumer Reports, *The Medicine Show*, 1974.

11. J. Katz, et al., "Sugar Consumption in Israeli Defense Forces Personnel," *Clin-Prev-Dent*, March-April 1991, No. 1392), pages 32-34.

12. A. Sheiham, "Why Free Sugars Consumption Should Be Below 15 kg Per Person Per Year in Industrialized Countries," *British Dent-Journal*, July 20, 1991, No. 171(2), pages 63-65.

13. A.J. Rugg-Gunn, "Diet and Dental Caries," *Dent-Update*, June 1990, No. 17(5), pages 198-201.

14. H. Graf, "Potential Cariogenicity of Low and High Sucrose Dietary Patterns," *Journal-Clinical-Periodontal*, November 1983, No. 10(6), pages 636-642.

15. A. Vrana, et al, "Sucrose Induced Hypertriglyceridaemia: Its Mechanisms and Metabolic Effects," *Czech-Med.*, 1982, No. 5(1), pages 9-15.

16. D. Sailer, "Does Sugar Play a Role in the Development of Gastroenterologic Diseases (Crohn Disease, Gallstones, Cancer)?", *Z-Ernahrungswiss*, 1990, No. 29 Suppl. 1, pages 39-44.

17. H. Forster, "Does Sugar Play a Role in the Development of Overweight?", *Z-Ernahrungswiss*, 1990, No. 29 Suppl. 1, pages 45-52.

18. G. Wolfram, "Is Sugar Involved in the Development of Cardiovascular Disease?", *Z-Ernahrungswiss*, 1990, No. 29 Suppl 1, pages 35-38.

19. J.B. Bristol, et al, "Sugar, Fat and the Risk of Colorectal Cancer," *British Medical Journal*, November 23, 1985, No. 291 (6507), pages 1467-1470.

20. B. Katschinski, et al, "Smoking and Sugar Intake are Separate but Interactive Risk Factors in Crohn's Disease," *Gut*, September 1988, No. 29(9), pages 1202-06.

21. K. Silkoff, et al, "Consumption of Refined Carbohydrate by Patients with Crohn's Disease in Tel-Aviv-Yafo," *Postgrad-Med-Journal*, December 1980, No. 56 (662), pages 842-846.

22. J.F. Riemann, S. Kolb, "Low Sugar and Fiber Rich Diet in Crohn Disease," *Fortschr-Med*, January 26, 1984, No. 102(4), pages 67-70.

23. L. Evans, et al, "Congenital Selective Malabsorption of Glucose and Galactose," *Journal-Pediatr-Gastroenterol-Nutr*, December 1985, No. 4(6), pages 878-886.

24. N.J. Blacklock, "Sucrose and Idiopathic Renal Stone," *Nutri-Health*, 1987, No. 5(1-2), pages 9-17.

25. M. Sorokin, "Hospital Morbidity in the Fiji Islands with Special Reference to the Saccharine Disease," *South African Medical Journal*, August 23, 1975, No. 49(36), pages 1481-1485.

26. S. Seely, D.F. Horrobin, "Diet and Breast Cancer: The Possible Connection with Sugar Consumption," *Med-Hypotheses*, July 1983, No. 11(3), pages 319-327.

27. A.M. Rossignol, H. Bonnlander, "Prevalence and Severity of the Premenstrual Syndrome. Effects of Foods and Beverages that are Sweet or High in Sugar Content," *Journal-Reprod-Med*, February 1991, No. 36(2), pages 131-36.

28. N.B. Kenepp, et al, "Fetal and Neonatal Hazards or Maternal Hydration With 5% Dextrose Before Caesarean Section," *Lancet*, May 22, 1982, No. 1(8282), pages 1150-1152.

29. S. Singhi, et al, "Intrapartum Infusion of Aqueous Glucose Solution, Transplacental Hyponatremia and Risk of Neonatal Jaundice," *British Journal of Obstetrics and Gynecology*, October 1984, No. 91(10), pages 1014-1018.

30. J. Glover, M. Sandilands, "Supplementation of Breastfeeding Infants and Weight Loss in Hospital," *Journal-Hum-Lact*, December 1990, No. 6(4), pages 163-166.

31. B. Guggenheim, E. Ben-Zur, "Fermentable Carbohydrates in Teething Preparations as a Cause of Caries in Small Children," *Schweiz-Med-Wochenschr*, February 13, 1982, No. 112(7), pages 232-234.

32. Wiley, Harvey W., **The History of a Crime Against the Food Law**, published by the author in Washington, D.C., 1929.

33. E.J. Feskins, et al, "Carbohydrate Intake and Body Mass Index in Relation to the Risk of Glucose Intolerance in an Elderly Population," *American Journal-Clinical-Nutr*, July 1991, No. 54(1), pages 136-140.

34. D.B. McWilliam, "The Practical Management of Glucose-Insulin Infusions in the Intensive Care Patient," *Intensive Care-Med*, 1980, No. 6(2), pages 133-135.

35. T.J. Maher, R.J. Wurtman, "Possible Neurologic Effects of Aspartame,"

Environealth-Perspective, November 1987, No. 75, pages 53-57.

36. A. Pinter, et al, "Comparative Studies on the Plaque Forming Effect of Sorbitol and Saccharose Containing Chocolate," *Dtsch-Zahnarztl-Z,* June 1978, No. 33(6), pages 418-420.

37. K.K. Park, et al, "Effect of Sorbitol Gum Chewing on Plaque PH Response After Ingesting Snacks Containing Predominantly Sucrose or Starch," *American Journal of Dentistry,* October 1990, No. 3(5), pages 185-191.

38. U. Keller, "The Sugar Substitutes Fructose and Sorbite: An Unnecessary Risk in Parental Nutrition," *Schweiz-Med-Wochenschr,* January 28, 1989, No. 119(4), pages 101-106.

39. D.E. Muller-Wiefel, et al, "Infusion-associated Kidney and Liver Failute in Undiagnosed Hereditary Fructose Intolerance," *Dtsch-Med-Wochenschr,* June 24, 1983, No. 108(25), pages 985-989.

Chapter 7

1. Geoffrey Cowley and John McCormick, "How Safe Is Our Food?", *Newsweek,* May 24, 1993, p. 52-55.

2. Ibid, p. 52.

3. A.M. Liebstein, M.D. and Neil L. Ehmki, "The Case for Vegetarianism," *American Mercury,* April 1950, p. 27.

4. Irvin Molotsky, "Chicken Inspection is Faulty," *New York Times,* May 13, 1987, p. C4.

5. "Safety of Meat Inspection Questioned," *Spectrum, The Wholistic News Magazine,* January/February 1992, p. 6.

6. "Nationline," *USA Today,* May 28, 1993, p. 3A.

7. *Spectrum,* p. 6.

8. *Newsweek,* p. 52.

9. C.A. Ryan et al., "Escherichia coli 0157:H7 diarrhea in a nursing home: clinical epidemiological and pathological findings," *J. Infec. Dis.,* October 1986, 154(4), p. 631-8.

10. Rick Weiss, "Are Fast Food Burgers Safe To Eat?", *Health,* May/June 1993, p. 14.

11. *Newsweek,* p. 53.

12. Guess What's Coming to Dinner — Contaminants in Our Food, Americans for Safe Food, Center for Science in the Public Interest, March 1987, p. 14.

13. B. Rowe et al., "Salmonella ealing infections associated with dried milk," *Lancet,* October 17, 1987 2(8564), p. 900-3.

14. K.C. Spitalny et al., "Salmonellosis outbreak in a Vermont hospital," *South Med. J.,* February 1984 77(2), p. 168-72.

15. G.R. Istre et al., "Campylobacter enteritis associated with undercooked barbecued chicken," *Amer. J. Public Health*, November 1984 74(11), p. 1265-7.

16. *Newsweek*, p. 52.

17. Ibid, p. 54.

18. B. Schwartz et al., "Association of sporadic listeriosis with consumption of uncooked hotdogs and undercooked chicken," *Lancet*, October 1, 1988 2(8614), p. 779-82.

19. K.A. Glass and M.P. Doyle, "Fate of listeria monocytogenes in processed meat products during refrigerated storage," *Appl. Environ. Microbiol.* (United States), June 1989 55(6), p. 1565-9.

20. S.M. Landry et al., "Trichinosis: common source outbreak related to commercial pork," *South Med. J.*, April 1992 85(4), p. 428-9.

21. Peter M. Schantz, "Trichinosis in the United States, 1985: Increase in Cases Attributed to Numerous Common-Source Outbreaks," *The Journal of Infectious Diseases*, 136, no. 5, November 1977, p. 712-15.

22. "EPA Decides Carcinogen is OK for Eggs and Chicken," *Vegetarian Times*, July 1984.

23. "Is Our Food Safe?", *Spectrum, The Wholistic News* Magazine, May/June 1991, p. 11.

24. Michael Hansen, "Animal Drugs in Our Food Supply," *NYCAP News*, New York Coalition for Alternatives to Pesticides, Late Summer 1992, p. 31.

25. *New England Journal of Medicine*, September 6, 1984.

26. Suzanne D. Caudry and Vilma A. Stanisick, "Incidence of antibiotic-resistant escherichia coli associated with frozen chicken carcasses and characterization of conjugative R plasmids derived from such strains," *Antimicrobial Agents and Chemotherapy*, December 1979, p. 701.

27. "Antibiotics Can Lead to Tainted Meat," *USA Today*, September 6, 1984, p. D1.

28. Bill Keller, "Ties to Human Illness Revive Move to Ban Medicated Feed," *New York Times*, September 9, 1984, p. 1.

29. "Chloramphenicol Use by Cattlemen Said to be Dangerous," *Vegetarian Times*, September 1984, p. 6.

30. David Bauman and Timothy Kenny, "Cattle Drug May Be Tied to Early Puberty," *USA Today*, December 5, 1984.

31. "Hormonal Time Bomb?", *Time*, August 2, 1971.

32. "Evidence Mounts Against DES," *USA Today*, December 7, 1984.

33. Hall, **Food for Naught.**

34. S.S. Epstein, "The Chemical Jungle: Today's Beef Industry," *Int. J. Health Serv.*, 1990, 20(2), p. 277-80.

35. "Is Our Food Safe?", *Spectrum*, May/June 1991, p. 11.

36. "Dangerous Chemicals in Meat," *Natural Living Newsletter, no. 40.*

37. Dan Fagin, "Cancer Causer: Study Shows DDT Residues Increase Risk,"

New York Newsday, April 21, 1993, p. 7.

38. Fred Zahradnik, "EPA Suppresses Rural Water Study," *The New Farm*, January 1984.

39. The Meat Sourcebook, *The American Meat Institute*, Chicago, 1960, p. 43.

40. D.A. Snowdon, R.L. Phillips and G.E. Fraser, "Meat Consumption and Fatal Ischemic Heart Disease," *Prev. Med.*, September 1984, 13(5), p. 490-500.

41. M. Mori and H. Miyake, "Dietary and Other Risk Factors of Ovarian Cancer Among Elderly Women," Jpn.J. *Cancer Res.*, September 1988, 79(9), p. 997-1004.

42. W.C. Willett, et al., "Relation of Meat, Fat, and Fiber Intake to the Risk of Colon Cancer in a Prospective Study Among Women," *N. Engl. J. Med.*, December 13, 1990, 323(24), p. 1664-72.

43. A.A. Nanji and S.W. French, "Relationship Between Pork Consumption and Cirrhosis," *Lancet*, March 23, 1985, 1(8430), p. 681-3.

44. J.T. Dwyer, "Health Aspects of Vegetarian Diets," *Am. J. Clin. Nutr.*, September 1988, 48(3 Suppl.), p. 712-38.

45. L.J. Beilin, et al., "Vegetarian Diet and Blood Pressure Levels: Incidental or Causal Association?", *Am J. Clin. Nutr.*, September 1988, 48 (3 Suppl.) p. 806-10.

46. "Vegetarians — Twice the Immune Punch," *Spectrum, The Wholistic News Magazine*, January/February 1992, p. 5.

Chapter 8

1. **Clearing the Air:** Preparing for a Smoke-Free Workplace, Alexander Hamilton Institute Inc., Maywood, N.J., 1993.

2. Kenneth A. Moore, "The High Cost of Smoking," *Business & Health*, Medical Economics Publishing, 1992, p. 11.

3. **Clearing the Air:** Preparing for a Smoke Free Workplace, p. 1.

4. **On the Air:** A Guide to Creating a Smoke-Free Workplace, American Lung Association, New York, N.Y., 1992, p. 8.

5. **Clearing the Air:** Preparing for a Smoke-Free Workplace, p. 2.

6. Kenneth A. Moore, "A look at Smoking in the Workplace," *Business & Health*, Medical Economics Publishing, 1992, p. 8.

7. **On the Air:** A Guide to Creating a Smoke-Free Workplace, p. 16.

8. Moore, "The High Cost of Smoking," p. 9.

9. **On the Air:** A Guide to Creating a Smoke-Free Workplace, p. 16.

10. Russell, M.A. Hamilton, "Cigarette Smoking; a Natural History of a Dependence Disorder," *British Journal of Medical Psychology*, (44), 1971.

11. Johnston, Lennox M., Tobacco Smoking and Nicotine, *Lancet*, December 19, 1942.

12. **On the Air:** A Guide to Creating a Smoke-Free Workplace, p. 18.

13. Alcohol, *Health & Research World*, Vol. 15(1), 1991, p. 91-96.

14. U.S. Department of Transportation's National Highway Traffic Safety Administration, Washington D.C., 1992.

15. Ibid.

16. R. Jenkins, et al, "A Six Year Longitudinal Study of the Occupational Consequences of Drinking Over 'Safe Limits' of Alcohol," *Br-J-Ind-Med*, May 1992, No. 49(5), pages 369-374.

17. R.G. Batey, et al, "Alcohol Consumption and the Risk of Cirrhosis," *Med-J-Aust*, March 16, 1992, No. 156(6), pages 413-416.

18. G. Corrao, et al, "Alcohol Consumption and Non-Cirrhotic Chronic Hepatitis: A Case Control Study," *Int-J-Epidemiol*, December 1991, No. 20(4), pages 1037-1042.

19. S. Shiomi, et al, "Effect of Drinking on the Outcome of Cirrhosis in Patients with Hepatitis B or C," *J-Gastroenterol-Hepatol*, May-June 1992, No. 7(3), pages 274-276.

20. H. Maier, et al, "Tobacco and Alcohol and the Risk of Head and Neck Cancer," *Clin-Investig*, March-April 1992, No. 70(3-4), pages 320-327.

21. S.Y. Choi, H. Kahyo, "Effect of Cigarette Smoking and Alcohol Consumption in the Aetiology of Cancer of the Oral Cavity, Pharynx and Larynx," *Int-J-Epidemiol*, December 1991, No. 20(4), pages 878-885.

22. E.V. Bandera, et al, "Alcohol Consumption and Lung Cancer in White Males," *Cancer-Causes-Control*, July 1992, No. 3(4), pages 361-369.

23. G.A. Kune, L. Vitetta, "Alcohol Consumption and the Etiology of Colorectal Cancer: A Review of the Scientific Evidence from 1957 to 1991," *Nutr-Cancer*, 1992, No. 18(2), pages 97-111.

24. M. Ferraroni, et al, "Alcohol and Breast Cancer Risk: A Case Control Study from Northern Italy," *Int-J-Epidemiol*, December 1991, No. 20(4), pages 859-864.

25. C. La Vecchia, et al, "Alcohol and Epithelial Overiarn Cancer," *J-Clin-Epidemiol*, September 1992, No. 45(9), pages 1025-1030.

26. V.J. Adesso, et al, "The Acute Effects of Alcohol on the Blood Pressure of Young, Normotensive Men," *Journal-Study-Alcohol*, September 1990, No. 51(5), pages 468-471.

27. J.S. Gill, et al, "Alcohol Consumption: A Risk Factor for Hemorrhagic and Non-Hemorrhagic Stroke," *American Journal of Medicine*, April 1991, No. 90(4), pages 489-497.

28. H. Loser, et al, "Alcohol in Pregnancy and Fetal Heart Damage," *Klin-Padiatr*, September-October 1992, No. 204(5), pages 335-339.

29. The President's Commission on Law Enforcement and Administration of Justice, Appendix I, **Task Force Report:** Drunkenness, 1967.

30. P.E. Bijur, et al, "Parental Alcohol Use, Problem Drinking, and Children's Injuries," *JAMA*, June 17, 1992, No. 267(23), pages 3166-3171.

31. McManamy, Margaret C., and Schube, Purcell G., "Caffeine Intoxication" *New England Journal of Medicine*, (215) 1936.

32. A.M. Rossignol, et al, "Tea and Premenstrual Syndrome in the People's Republic of China," *American Journal of Public Health*, January 1989, No. 79(1), pages 67-69.

33. A.M. Rossingnol, H. Bonnlander, "Caffeine-containing Beverages, Total Fluid Consumption and Premenstrual Syndrome," *American Journal of Public Health*, September 1990, No. 80(9), pages 1106-1110.

34. K.D. Lindsted, et al, "Coffee Consumption and Cause-Specific Mortality. Association With Age at Death and Compression of Mortality," *Journal-Clinical-Epidemiol*, July 1992, No. 45(7), pages 733-742.

35. *Science Digest*, June, 1973.

36. *Consumer Bulletin Annual*, 1972.

37. R.J. Mathew, W.H. Wilson, "Behavioral and Cerebrovascular Effects of Caffeine in Patients with Anxiety Disorders," *Acta-Psychiatr-Scand*, July 1990, No. 82(1), pages 17-22.

38. J.S. Walker, "Phenylpropanolamine Potentiates Caffeine Neurotoxicity in Rats," *Journal-Pharm-Sci*, December 1989, No. 78(12), pages 986-989.

39. M.A. Lee, et al, "Anxiogenic Effects of Caffeine on Panic and Depressed Patients," *American Journal of Psychiatry*, May 1988, No. 145(5), pages 632-635.

40. G.L. Clementz, J.W. Dailey, "Psychotropic Effects of Caffeine," *American Family Physician*, May 1988, No. 37(5), pages 167-172.

41. *The New York Post* (The Associated Press), February 3, 1976, p. 67.

42. B.G. Armstrong, et al, "Cigarette, Alcohol and Coffee Consumption and Spontaneous Abortion," *American Journal of Public Health*, January 1992, No. 82(1), pages 85-87.

43. M.A. Williams, et al, "Cigarettes, Coffee and Preterm Premature Rupture of the Membranes," *American Journal-Epidemiol*, April 15, 1992, No. 135(8), pages 895-903.

44. H.S. Salvador, B.J. Koos, "Effects of Regular and Decaffeinated Coffee on Fetal Breathing and Heart Rate," *American Journal of Obstetrics and Gynecology*, May 1989, No. 160 (5 Pt 1), pages 1043-1047.

45. J. Olsen, et al, "Coffee Consumption, Birthweight and Reproductive Failures," *Epidemiology*, September 1991, No. 2(5), pages 370-374.

46. S.G. Gilbert, et al, "Adverse Pregnancy Outcome in the Monkey (Macaca fascicularis) After Chronic Caffeine Exposure," *Journal-Pharmocol-Exp-Ther*, June 1988, No. 245(3), pages 1048-1053.

47. J.D. McGowan, et al, "Neonatal Withdrawal Symptoms After Chronic Maternal Ingestion of Caffeine," *South-Med-Journal*, September 1988, No. 81(9), pages 1092-1094.

48. C. Johansson, et al, "Coffee Drinking: A Minor Risk Factor for Bone Loss and Fractures," *Age-Aging*, January 1992, No. 21(1), pages 20-26.

49. D.P. Kiel, et al, "Caffeine and the Risk of Hip Fracture: The Framingham Study," *American Journal-Epidemiology*, October 1990, No. 132(4), pages 675-684.

50. J.L. Lyon, et al, "Coffee Consumption and the Risk of Cancer of the Exocrine

Pancreas: A Case-Control Study in a Low-Risk Population," *Epidemiology*, March 1992, No. 3(2), pages 164-170.

51. M. Jarebinski, et al, "Evaluation of the Association of Cancer of the Esophagus, Stomach and Colon with Habits of Patients," *Vojnosanit-Pregl*, January-February 1992, No. 49(1), pages 19-24.

52. C.W. Welsch, J.V. DeHoog, "Influence of Caffeine Consumption on 7, 12-Dimethylbenz (a) anthracene-Induced Mammary Gland Tumorigenesis in Female Rats Fed a Chemically Defined Diet Containing Standards and High Levels of Unsaturated Fat," *Cancer Research*, April 15, 1988, No. 48(8), pages 2074-2077.

53. A.A. Rizzo, et al, "Effects of Caffeine Withdrawal on Motor Performance and Heart Rate Changes," *International Journal of Psychophysiology*, March 1988, No. 6(1), pages 9-14.

54. J.R. Hughes, et al, "Caffeine Self-Administration, Withdrawal and Adverse Effects Among Coffee Drinkers," *Arch-Gen-Psychiatry*, July 1991, No. 48(7), pages 611-617.

55. M.J. Shirlow, et al, "Caffeine Consumption and Blood Pressure: An Epidemiological Study," *International Journal of Epidemiology*, March 1988, No. 17(1), pages 90-97.

Chapter 9

1. U.S. Department of Commerce, 1970.

2. Winter, Ruth, *Consumer's Dictionary of Cosmetic Ingredients*, New York, Crown Publishers, Inc., 1974.

3. Wells, F.V., and Lubowe, Irwin, **Cosmetics and the Skin**, New York, Van Nostrand, 1964.

4. U.S. Food and Drug Administration, 1974.

5. *Consumer Reports*, Aerosols: The Medical Cost of Convenience, May, 1974.

6. "Paraben Allergy — A Cause of Intractable Dermatitis," *Journal of the American Medical Association*, Vol. 204, No. 10, June 3, 1968.

7. Brodeur, Paul, **Asbestos and Enzymes**, New York, Ballantine Books, 1972.

8. U.S. F.D.A., 1974.

9. *Consumer Reports*, ibid.

10. Stabile, Toni, **Cosmetics:** The Great American Skin Game, Ballantine, New York, 1973.

11. "Chemical Depilatories," *Consumers' Research Magazine*, January, 1974.

Chapter 10

1. W.M. Harrison, et al., "MAIOs and Hypertensive Crises: The Role of OTC

Drugs," *J. Clin. Psychiatry*, February 1989, 50(2), p. 64-65.

2. Ibid.

3. "Adverse Reactions to Over-the-counter analgesics: an Epidemiological Evaluation," Agents. Actions. Suppl., 1988, 25, p. 21-31.

4. Ibid.

5. P.P. Lamy, "Over the Counter Medication: The Drug Interactions We Overlook," *J. Am. Geriatr. Soc.*, November 1982, 30 (11 Suppl). ps. 69-75.

6. Ibid.

7. Ibid.

8. Ibid.

9. *New York Times*, January 28, 1976, p. 1.

10. Competitive Problems in the Drug Industry, Hearings Before the Subcommittee on Monopoly, Senate Select Committee on Small Business, 90th through 93rd Congress (1967-1974).

11. Louis S. Goodman and A. Gilman, editors, **Pharmacological Basis of Therapeutics**, New York and London, 1965.

12. **New York Times Encyclopedic Almanac**, 1975.

13. J.K. French et al., "Milk Alkali Syndrome Following Over-the-Counter Antacid Self-Medication," *N. Z. Med. J.*, May 14, 1986, 99(801), p. 322-3.

14. The Boston Collaborative Drug Surveillance Program, Boston University Medical Center, 1975.

15. Richard Burach, with Fred J. Fox, **The New Handbook of Prescription Drugs,** Ballantine Books, New York, 1975.

16. W.E. Thornton, "Sleep aids and Sedatives," *JACEP*, September 1977, 6(9), p. 408-12.

17. Ibid.

18. The Planned Parenthood Federation of America, **Contraceptives Study,** 1975

19. *Consumer Reports*, Serc: A Dizzying Story of Vertigo in the F.D.A., March 1973.

Reading List

Global Warming

Robert Cooke, "Life in a Greenhouse," *New York Newsday*, September 13, 1988, Part III, p. 1.

Lani Sinclair, **Changing Climate:** A Guide to the Greenhouse Effect, World Resources Institute, Washington D.C.

Cooling the Greenhouse: Vital First Steps to Combat Global Warming, Natural Resources Defense Council, Washington D.C.

Policy Options for Stabilizing Global Climate: Draft Report to Congress, U.S. Environmental Protection Agency, Washington, D.C.

The Potential Effects of Global Warming on the United States, Draft Report to Congress (Executive Summary), U.S. Environmental Protection Agency, Washington D.C.

The Ozone Layer

Ellen Ruppel Shell, "Watch This Space," *Omni*, August 1987.

Washington Post Wire Service, "97% Drop in Ozone Recorded Over Antarctica," *The Star Ledger*, October 28, 1987, p. 21.

Natural Resources Defense Council, "Ozone Depletion Worsens," *Newsline*, p. 1.

Dick Russell, "The Endless Simmer," *In These Times*, January 11, 1989, p. 10.

"Can We Repair the Sky?", Reprint from Consumer Reports, Mount Vernon, New York.

Protecting the Ozone Layer: What You Can Do, Environmental Defense Fund, New York, N.Y.

Saving the Ozone Layer: A Citizen Action Guide, Natural Resources Defense Council, New York, N.Y.

Stones in a Glass House — CFC's and Ozone Depletion, Investor Responsibility Research Center, Washington, D.C.

Acid Rain

National Audubon Society, "Monthly Report of pH Readings," *Citizen's Acid Rain Monitoring Network*, January 1988.

Air Pollution, Acid Rain and the Future of the Forest, World Watch Institute, Washington, D.C.

Trends in the Quality of the Nation's Air, U.S. Environmental Protection Agency, Washington D.C.

Water Pollution

"Cleanup of A Pure River," *East/West*, June 1987, p. 13.

Larry J. Brown and Deborah Allen, "Toxic Waste and Citizen Action," *Science for the People*, July/August 1983, p. 6.

K. Barton, "Fish Cancer," *Environment*, November 1983, p. 24.

Kuchenberg, "Measuring the Health of the Ecosystem," *Environment*, March 1985, p. 32.

Tim Johnson, "The Poisoned Turtle," *Daybreak*, Summer 1988, p. 25.

Zev Remba, "Beyond Water Wasteland," *Clean Water Action News*, Summer 1987.

William K. Burke, "An Effluent Community Worries . . ." *In These Times*, April 12, 1989, p. 8.

Dick Thompson, "The Greening of the U.S.S.R.," *Time*, January 2, 1989, p. 68.

Jane McCarthy, "Fishy Mystery of Dead Sea on N.J. Shore," *New York Post*, August 29, 1988, p. 14.

Dick Thompson, "Stains on the White Continent," *Time*, February 20, 1989, p. 77.

"Today's Robber Barons Despoil the Environment," *In These Times*, April 12, 1989, p. 14.

Michael D. Lemonick, "The Two Alaskas," *Time*, April 17, 1989, p. 56.

Jonathan King, "Troubled Water," Rodale's Practical Homeowner, January 1987.

John Langone, "A Stinking Mess," *Time*, January 2, 1989, p. 47.

Lisa Lefferts and Stephen Schmidt, "Water: Safe to Swallow?", *Nutrition Action Health Letter*, November 1988, p.5.

J. Sibbison, "The Battle to Ban Fluorides," *Bestways*, December 1982, p. 60.

Ken Geiser and Gerry Waneck, "PCB's and Warren County," *Science for the People*, July/August 1983, p. 13.

J. Sibbison, "Ground Water Contamination," *Bestways*, October 1985.

Lee Steppacher and Tara Gallagher, "Natural Resources," *Environment*, May 1988.

The Chesapeake Bay Foundation Homeowner's Series: **Water Conservation, Household Hazardous Waste,** Detergents, The Chesapeake Bay Foundation, Annapolis, Maryland.

A Citizen's Guide to River Conservation, The Conservation Foundation, Washington D.C.

Danger On Tap, The Government's Failure to Enforce the Federal Safe Drinking Water Act, National Wildlife Foundation, Washington D.C.

Drinking Water — A Community Action Guide, Concern Inc., Washington D.C.

Raymond Gabler, Is Your Water Safe to Drink?, *Consumer Reports.*

Waste Disposal

J.W. Jeffery, "The Collapse of Nuclear Economic," *The Ecologist*, January/February 1988, p. 9.

Peter Bunyard, "The Myth of France's Cheap Nuclear Electricity," *Ecology*, January/February 1988, p. 4.

Mark Miller, "Not So Bad After All?" *Newsweek*, July 25, 1988, p. 65.

Jean Miller, "Major Radium Dump Found in New York City," *RWC Waste Paper*, Fall 1988, p. 3.

Danger Downwind: A Report on the Release of Billions of Pounds of Toxic Air Pollutants, National Wildlife Federation, Washington, D.C.

"Superfund: Looking Back, Looking Ahead," *EPA Journal*, January/February 1987.

Tom Krattenmaker, "Warning Sent to Shore Polluters," *Daily Record*, Morris County N.J., April 23, 1989, p. B12.

"Plastics Tax Slated for Senate Vote," *Daily Record*, Morris County N.J., April 23, 1989.

E. Majnuson, "A Problem that Cannot Be Buried," *Time*, October 14, 1985, p. 76.

"Right Train, Wrong Track: New Report on EPA's Mismanagement of Superfund," *NRDC Newsline*, July/August 1988, p. 1.

Chapter 3

J. Laseter, "Chlorinated Hydrocarbon Pesticides in Environmentally Sensitive Patients," *Clinical Ecology*, Vol. 11, No. 1, Fall 1983, p. 3.

"National Health Council Report," An Assessment of Health Risk of Seven Pesticides Used for Termite Control 9, National Academy Press, Washington, D.C., 1992.

K. Johnson, "Equity in Hazard Management," Environment, November 1982, p. 29.

T. Goldfarb and D. Wartenberg, "Fighting Pesticides on Long Island," *Science for the People*, January/February 1983, p. 18.

J. Eggington, "Temik Troubles Move South," *Audubon*, May 1993.

Rick McGuire, "Dioxin Pollution Called Pervasive," *Medical Tribune*, December 24, 1986, p. 5.

Carol Van Strum, "A Bitter Fog," *East/West Journal*, July 1983, p. 48.

Janet Hathaway, "Eating Wisely Gets Harder All the Time," *Los Angeles Times*, October 8, 1987.

J. Sibbison, "Why We're Still Eating Pesticides," *Bestways*, December 1982, p. 30.

Natural Resources Defense Council, *Pesticides in Food*, March 15, 1984.

Sheila Kaplan, "The Food Chain Gang," *Common Cause Magazine*, September/October 1987.

Margaret Carlson, "Do You Care To Eat A Peach?", *Time*, March 27, 1989, p. 24.

Diffusing the Toxic Threat: Controlling Pesticides and Industrial Wastes, Worldwatch Institute, Washington D.C.

Roger Yepsen Jr., *Encyclopedia of Natural Insect and Disease Control*, Rodale Press, Emmaus, PA.

Chapter 4

"The FDA and Nitrite," a case study of violations of the Food, Drug and Cosmetic Act with respect to a particular food additive, mimeographed report by Dale Hattis, Dept. of Genetics, Stanford University School of Medicine, April 25, 1972, sponsored and distributed by the Environmental Defense Fund, Washington, D.C.

"How Sodium Nitrite Can Affect Your Health," report by Michael F. Jacobson, Ph.D., Center for Science in the Public Interest, 1779 Church Street, N.W., Washington, D.C. 20036, February 1973.

"Regulation of Food Additives — Nitrites and Nitrates," 19th report of the Committee on Government Operations, House of Representatives, Aug. 15, 1972, based on a study by the Intergovernmental Relations Subcommittee (a Fountain committee report).

"Chemicals and the Future of Man," hearings before the Subcommittee on

Executive Reorganization and Government Research of the Committee on Government Operations, U.S. Senate, 92nd Congress, April 6 and 7, 1971 (chaired by Sen. Abraham A. Ribicoff).

"Nutrition and Human Needs — Food Additives," Parts 4A, 4B and 4C, hearings before the Select Committee on Nutrition and Human Needs, U.S. Senate, 92nd Congress, 19, 20, 21, 1972 (chaired by Sen. Gaylord Nelson).

"Regulation of Food Additives and Medicated Animal Feeds," hearings before a subcommittee of the Committee on Government Operations, House of Representatives, 92nd Congress, March 16, 17, 18, 29 and 30, 1971 (Fountain).

"The Toxic Substances Control Act of 1971 and Amendment," hearings on S. 1478 before the Subcommittee on the Environment of the Committee on Commerce, U.S. Senate, 92nd Congress, 1st session, Aug. 3, 4, 5, Oct. 4 and Nov. 5, 1971.

Chapter 5

Food and Water Inc., "Comments on the Food Marketing Institute's Report on Food Irradiation," Denville, N.J., July 15, 1988.

C. Bhaskaram and G. Sadasivan, "Effects of Feeding Irradiated Wheat To Malnourished Children," *Amer. J. Clin. Nutr.*, Vol. 28, 1975, p. 130.

Ken Terry, "Why Is the DOE for Food Irradiation," *The Nation*, February 1987, p. 143.

"New Push for Food Irradiation," *NYCAP News* (New York Coalition for Alternatives to Pesticides, Albany, N.Y.), Early Spring 1993, p. 29.

Dr. Yin, "Safety Evaluation of Irradiated Foods in China: A Condensed Report," *Biomed. Environ. Sci.*, March 1989, 2(1), p. 1-6.

A. Miller and P.H. Jensen, "Measurements of Induced Radioactivity in Electron and Photon-Irradiated Beef," *Int. J. Rad. Appl. Instrum.*, 1987, 38(7), p. 507-12.

Resources

Dr. Wyrth Post Baker
4701 Willard Avenue
Chevy Chase, Maryland 20815
(301) 656-8940

Dr. Steven J. Bock
Rhinebeck Health Center
108 Montgomery Street
Rhinebeck, New York 12572
(914) 876-7082

Dr. Jennifer Brett
988 Nichols Avenue
Stratford, Connecticut
(203) 377-1525

Dr. Dorothy Calbrese
655 Camino de los Mares #126
San Clemente, California 92673
(714) 240-7178

Dr. Robert Cathcart
(415) 949-2822

Dr. I-Tsu Chao
1641 East 18th Street
Brooklyn, New York 11229
(718) 998-3331

Dr. Charles H. Farr
10101 S. Western
Oklahoma City, Oklahoma 73139
(405) 691-1112

Dr. Martin Feldman
132 East 76th Street
New York, New York 10016
(212) 213-3337

Dr. Pannathpur Jayalakshmi
6366 Sherwood Road
Philadelphia, Pennsylvania 19151
(215) 473-4226

Dr. Kirk Morgan
9105 U.S. Highway 42
Prospect, Kentucky 40059
(502) 228-0156

Dr. Louis Parrish
242 East 72nd, Suite 1E
New York, New York 10021
(212) 737-3636

Dr. William Philpott
17171 S.E. 29th Street
Choctaw, Oklahoma 73020
(405) 390-3009

Also by Gary Null . . .

"**E**very person takes his or her own journey in life," says Gary Null, "and must ultimately be their own guide. Tens of thousands of listeners have let me know that after doing therapy and group-work in the 1980s, they are now interested in self-directed change. This book asks pertinent questions that lead readers to consolidate their gains and move forward to a more fulfilling life."

You can become who you were meant to be—happy, productive and functional on all levels at all times. Taking that step into a brighter tomorrow means integrating what you've learned about mental, physical, spiritual and emotional health. Here famed health expert and media personality Gary Null presents a roundup of the latest and best information on achieving personal fulfillment and offers the keys to transformational change.

Based on tens of thousands of inquiries from people who listen to his radio show, this book helps you identify your true needs, discover what is meaningful in your life and remove obstacles to self-directed change. Presented in interactive format, *Change Your Life Now* asks you the right questions to clarify what makes you happy and how you can get it. It brings you a clear, organized way to find your own answers.

Code 2905 (6x9, 180 pp.) $9.95

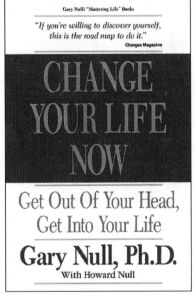

Gary Null's "Mastering Life" Books

"If you're willing to discover yourself, this is the road map to do it."
Changes Magazine

CHANGE YOUR LIFE NOW

Get Out Of Your Head, Get Into Your Life

Gary Null, Ph.D.
With Howard Null

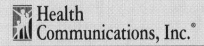

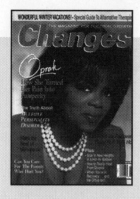